JN328303

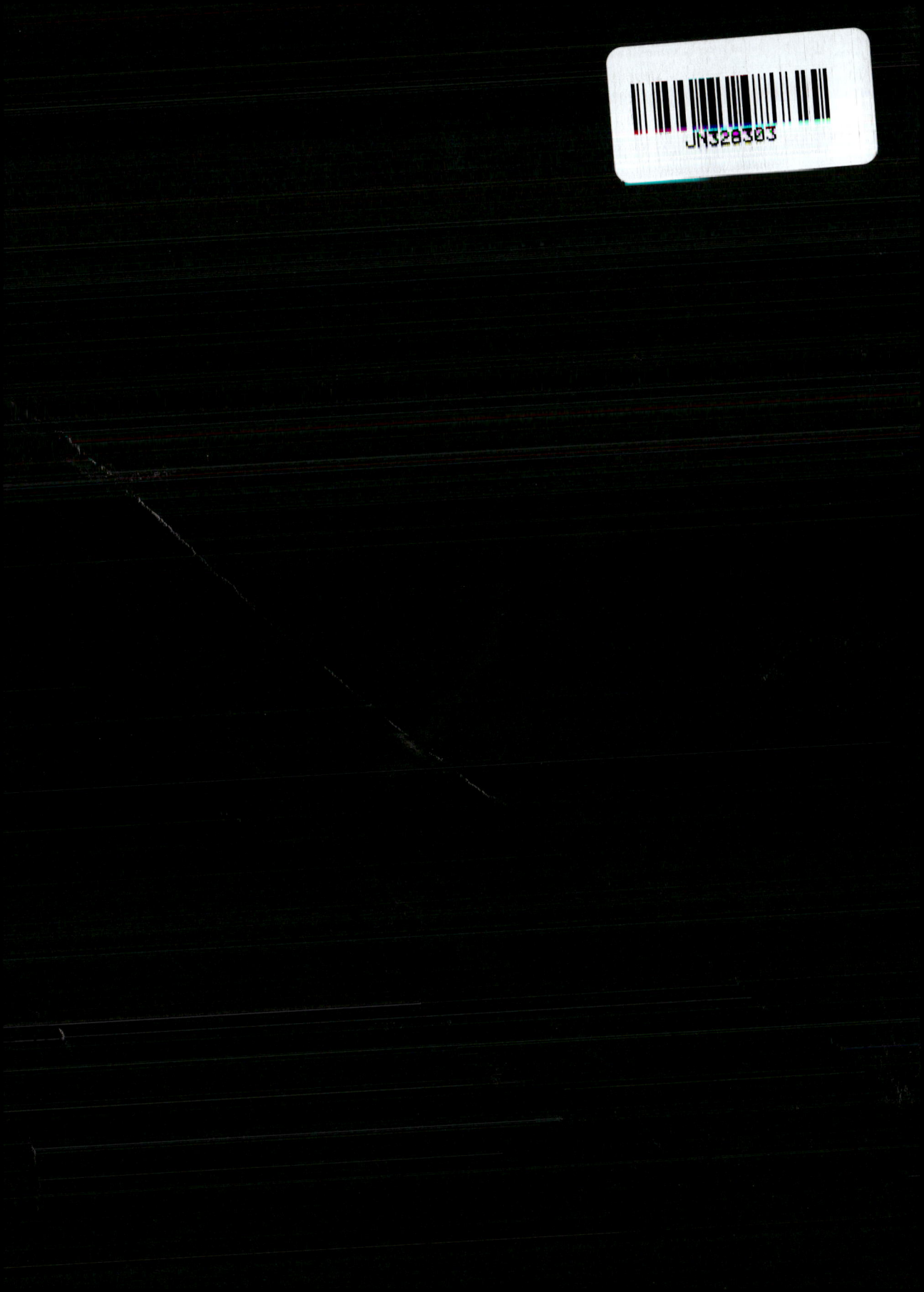

CT・MRI 解体新書

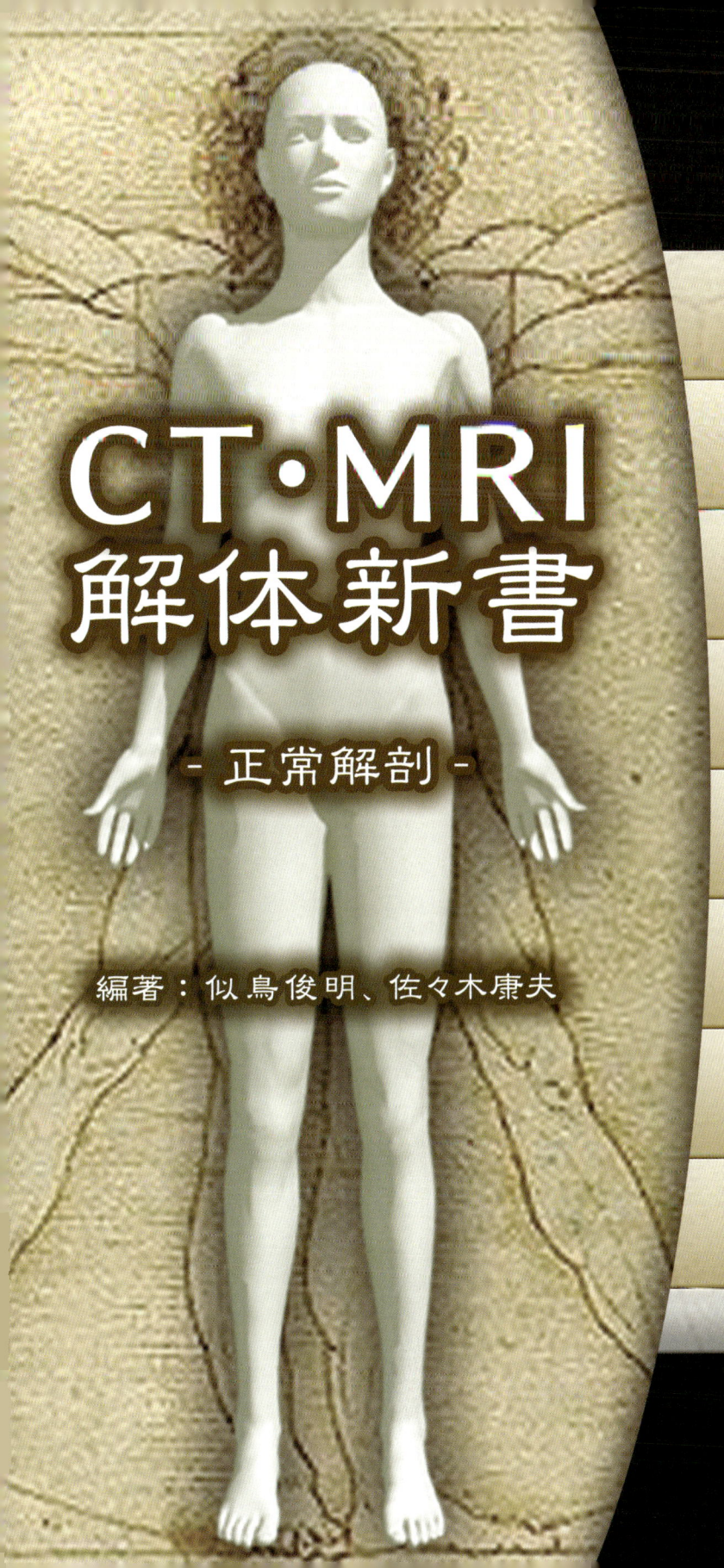

- 正常解剖 -

編著：似鳥俊明、佐々木康夫

Interactive CT and MRI Anatomy

- 頭部 Head
- 頭頸部 Neck
- 脊椎 Spine
- 胸部 Chest
- 腹部 Abdomen
- 骨盤（男性）Pelvis（Male）
- 骨盤（女性）Pelvis（Female）
- 四肢 Limbs
- Index

LibroScience

【編　著】　似鳥　俊明　（杏林大学医学部・放射線科 前教授）
　　　　　　佐々木 康夫　（岩手県立中央病院・放射線診断科長）

【著】　　　村上　清寿　（杏林大学医学部・放射線科）
　　　　　　林　　真弘　（杏林大学医学部・放射線科）

【執筆協力】　関澤　琢郎　（岩手県立中央病院・放射線診断科）
　　　　　　中山　　学　（岩手県立中央病院・放射線診断科）
　　　　　　及川　朋美　（岩手県立中央病院・放射線診断科）
　　　　　　小林　邦典　（杏林大学医学部付属病院・放射線部）

序

　この少しユニークな解剖学書の読者対象は極めて広い。医学部、保健学部などの学生、研修医、放射線技師、検査技師、看護師、そしてすべての医師が読者対象である。放射線科画像診断専門医も想定されている。現在の医療は極めて間口が広くかつ奥が深い。学びつつある者には目標が見えがたく、専門家にとってかつては広く学んだ専門外知識の保持が容易でない。医療の現場では互いの基本常識の解離が思わぬトラブルを招く。専門と専門の狭間にリスクが潜む。本書で掲載したものは、現在の医療でもはや欠くことのできないCT、MRIを中心とした画像医学の必須項目である。医療を学ぶすべての学生の目標点であり、すべての医療人が常識として常に保ちたいレベルである。

　本書の表紙、中扉の"ウィトルウィウスVitruvius的人体図"は、調和のとれた人体と神殿とをこのうえなく賛美した古代ローマ建築家の思想をダ・ヴィンチが視覚化したものである。調和の上に確立された専門性の象徴として用いた。

　巷間電子書籍が大いに注目されている。多くは紙媒体の書籍をPDFに置き換えたものであるが、我々はこれまでの電子書籍を超えた体験ができるiPhone用のアプリケーションを同時に開発し、ゲーム感覚で基本画像解剖を身につけることができるよう工夫した。書籍版、アプリ版ともにセルフチェックができる体裁であり、気軽に繰り返し学習、知識の確認をしてみてほしい。

　本企画は2010年春になされた。医療過疎化の中で健闘する岩手県の研修医たちを巻き込み、上記の思いを発信しようと作業を進めていたが、大きな災害が起こり頓挫しかけた。2011年3月の大震災・大津波で根底から揺すぶられて至った思い"ここですべきはすべての基本の総点検"……企画趣旨との符合に気付き、色合いをさらに明確にさせての作業再開で完成できたことを、全国からの支援に対する感謝の思いと共に付記したい。

2011年12月

似鳥 俊明、佐々木 康夫

Contents

頭　部 Head — 1

頭頸部 Neck — 21

脊　椎 Spine — 33

胸　部 Chest — 45

腹　部 Abdomen — 71

骨盤（男性）Pelvis (Male) — 93

骨盤（女性）Pelvis (Female) — 97

四　肢 Limbs — 103

    肩 Shoulder — 104

    肘 Elbow — 108

    手 Hand — 112

    股 Hip — 117

    膝 Knee — 120

    足 Foot — 124

Index — 131

参考図

1. 脳室の構造 ——————————————————————— 6
2. Willis動脈輪 ——————————————————————— 20
3. 脳の栄養動脈 —————————————————————— 32
4. 脊髄縦断像、および環椎と軸椎の関係 ———————————— 38
5. 肺区域とその名称 ———————————————————— 58
6. アメリカ心臓協会（AHA）による冠動脈セグメント ——————— 69
7. 体幹の動脈と静脈 ———————————————————— 70
8. 膵臓の脈管系 —————————————————————— 77
9. 肝区域 ————————————————————————— 78
10. 肝臓の脈管系と胆嚢・胆管との関係 ————————————— 83
11. 門脈系 ————————————————————————— 88
12. 腹腔動脈の枝 —————————————————————— 91
13. 小腸の血管支配 ————————————————————— 91
14. 大腸の血管支配 ————————————————————— 92
15. 上腸間膜動脈と下腸間膜動脈の枝 —————————————— 92
16. 大腿部の動静脈・神経の走行と大腿動静脈へのカテーテル刺入部位 — 96
17. 上肢・下肢の動脈 ———————————————————— 128
18. 上肢・下肢の静脈 ———————————————————— 129

v

本書の構成

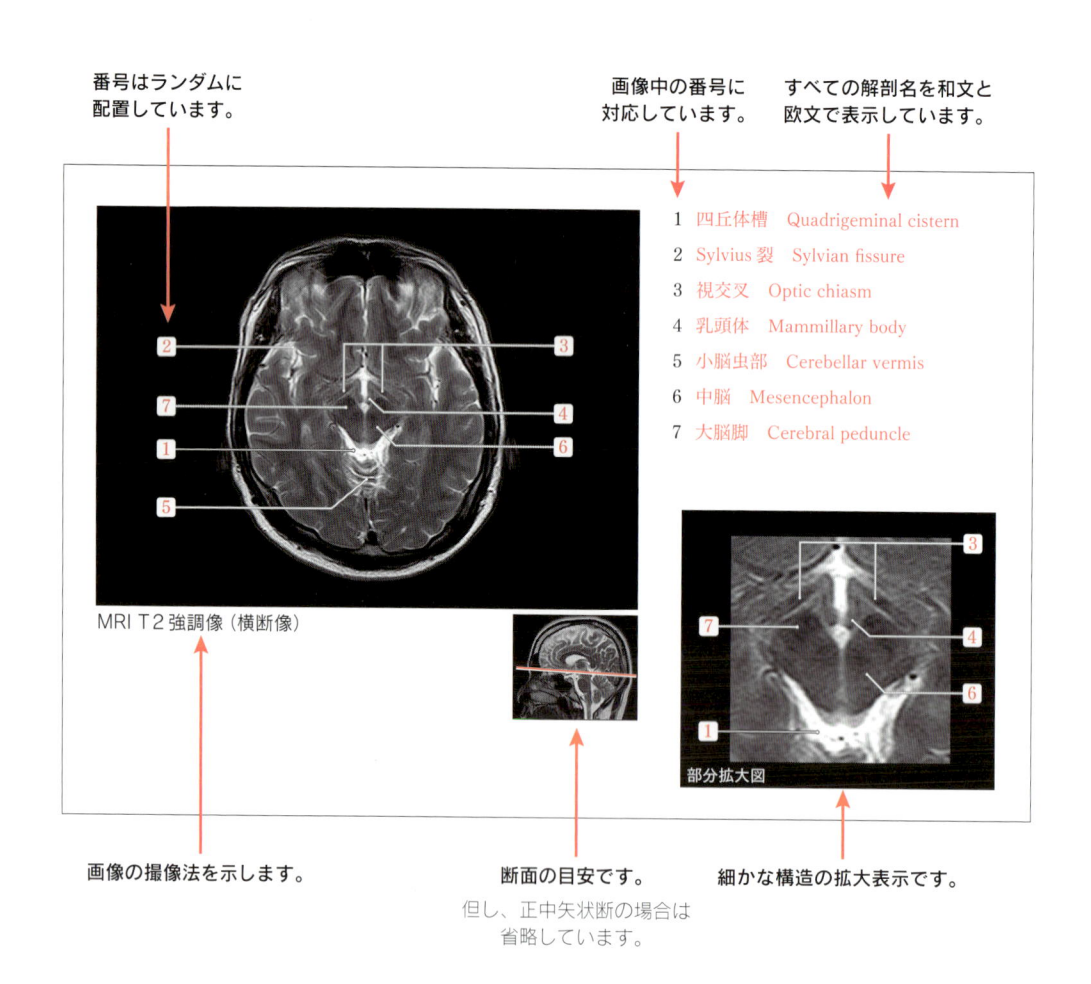

番号はランダムに配置しています。

画像中の番号に対応しています。

すべての解剖名を和文と欧文で表示しています。

1 四丘体槽　Quadrigeminal cistern
2 Sylvius裂　Sylvian fissure
3 視交叉　Optic chiasm
4 乳頭体　Mammillary body
5 小脳虫部　Cerebellar vermis
6 中脳　Mesencephalon
7 大脳脚　Cerebral peduncle

MRI T2強調像（横断像）

画像の撮像法を示します。

断面の目安です。
但し、正中矢状断の場合は省略しています。

部分拡大図

細かな構造の拡大表示です。

本書の使い方

付録の赤シートで解剖名や数字を隠してセルフチェックすることができます。

使い方 ①：画像中の番号を赤シートで隠す

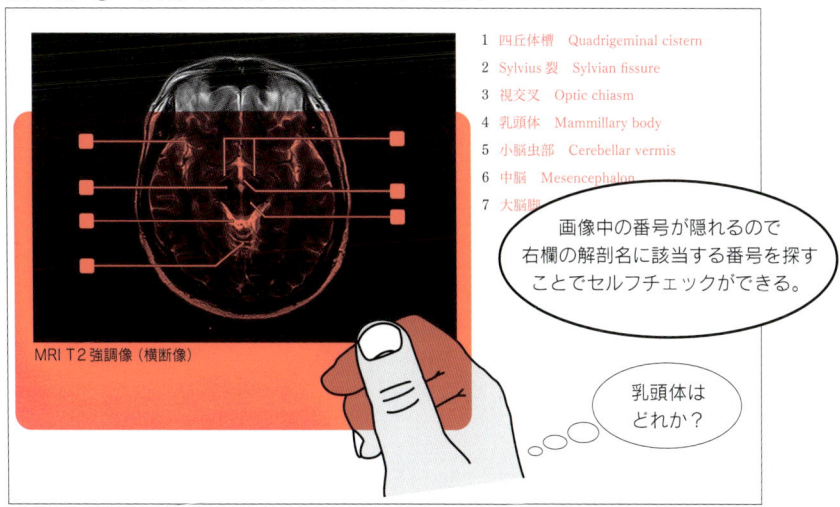

1 四丘体槽　Quadrigeminal cistern
2 Sylvius 裂　Sylvian fissure
3 視交叉　Optic chiasm
4 乳頭体　Mammillary body
5 小脳虫部　Cerebellar vermis
6 中脳　Mesencephalon
7 大脳脚

MRI T2強調像（横断像）

画像中の番号が隠れるので右欄の解剖名に該当する番号を探すことでセルフチェックができる。

乳頭体はどれか？

使い方 ②：解剖名を赤シートで隠す

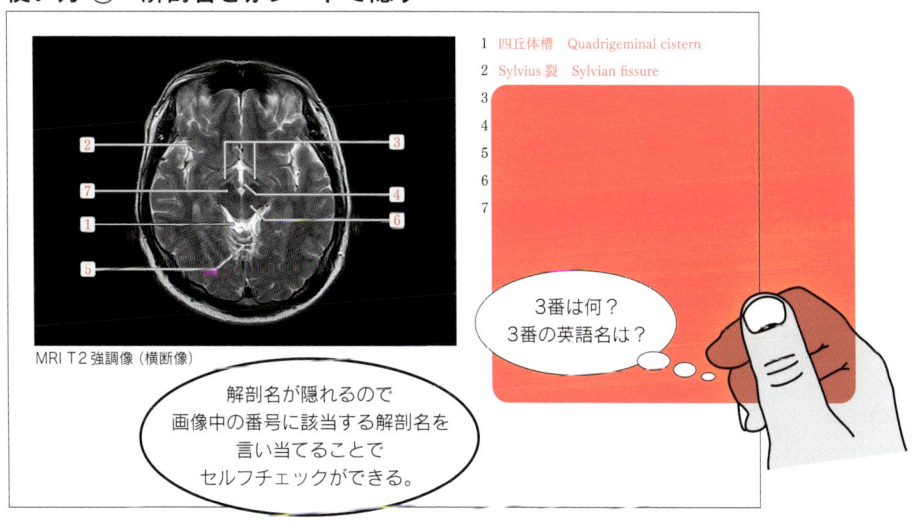

1 四丘体槽　Quadrigeminal cistern
2 Sylvius 裂　Sylvian fissure
3
4
5
6
7

MRI T2強調像（横断像）

解剖名が隠れるので画像中の番号に該当する解剖名を言い当てることでセルフチェックができる。

3番は何？
3番の英語名は？

CT・MRI 解体新書

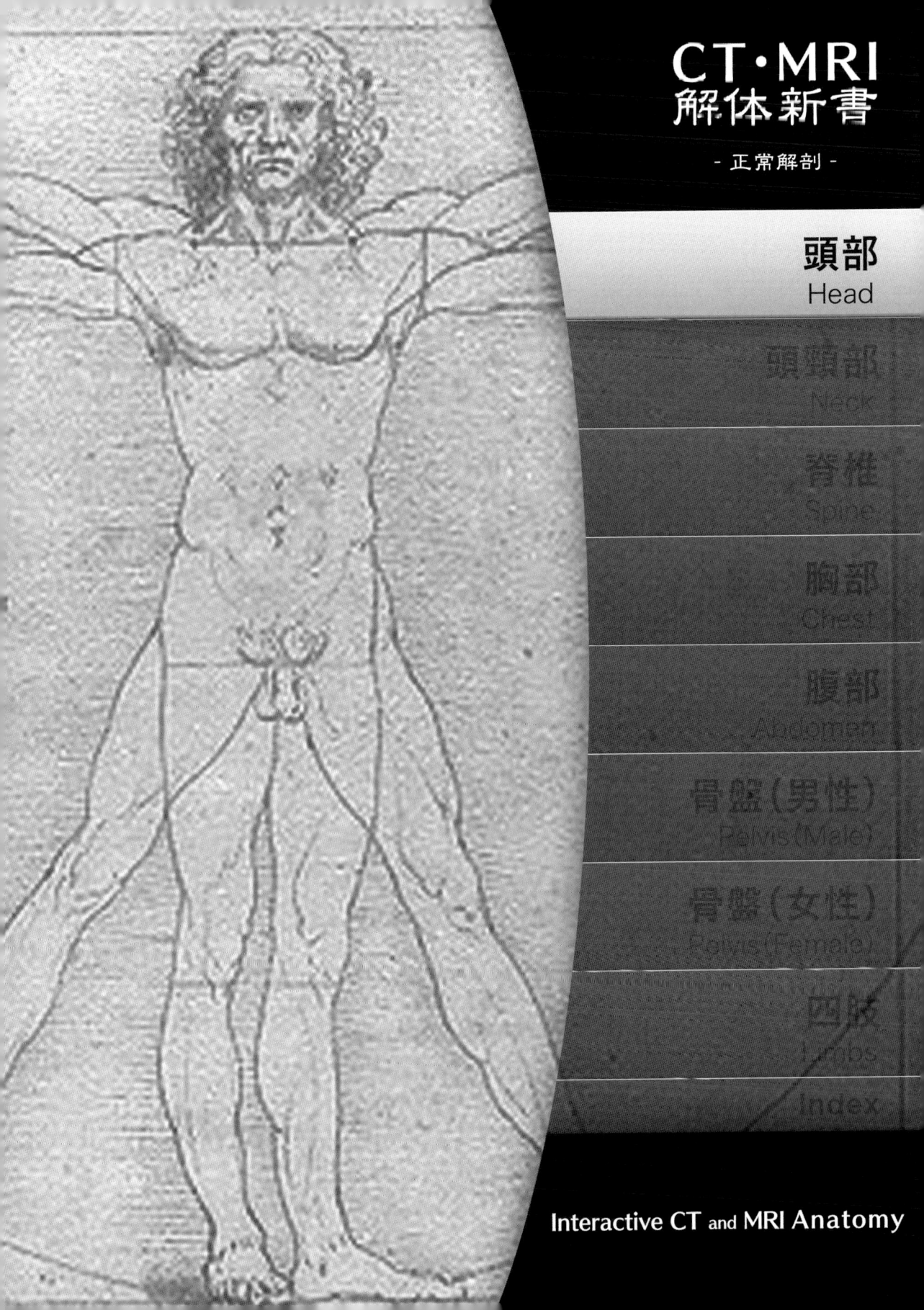

- 正常解剖 -

頭部
Head

頭頸部
Neck

脊椎
Spine

胸部
Chest

腹部
Abdomen

骨盤(男性)
Pelvis (Male)

骨盤(女性)
Pelvis (Female)

四肢
Limbs

Index

Interactive CT and MRI Anatomy

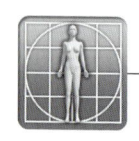

頭部
Head

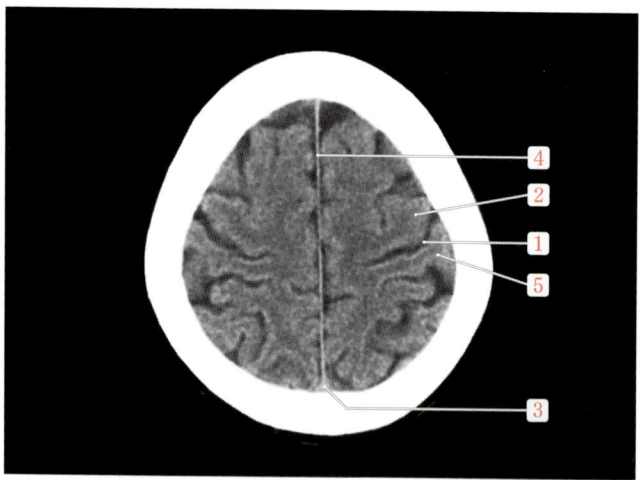

単純CT（横断像）

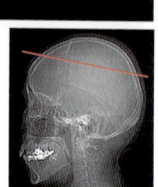

1 中心溝　Central sulcus
2 中心前回　Precentral gyrus
3 上矢状静脈洞　Superior sagittal sinus
4 大脳鎌　Falx cerebri
5 中心後回　Postcentral gyrus

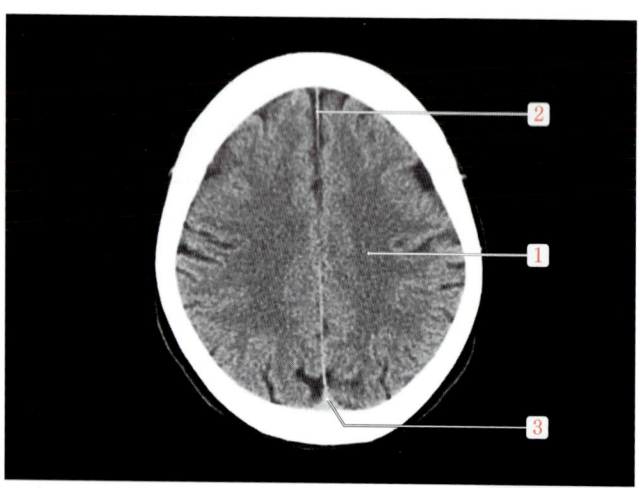

単純CT（横断像）

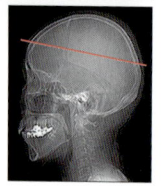

1 半卵円中心　Centrum semiovale
2 大脳鎌　Falx cerebri
3 上矢状静脈洞　Superior sagittal sinus

単純CT（横断像）

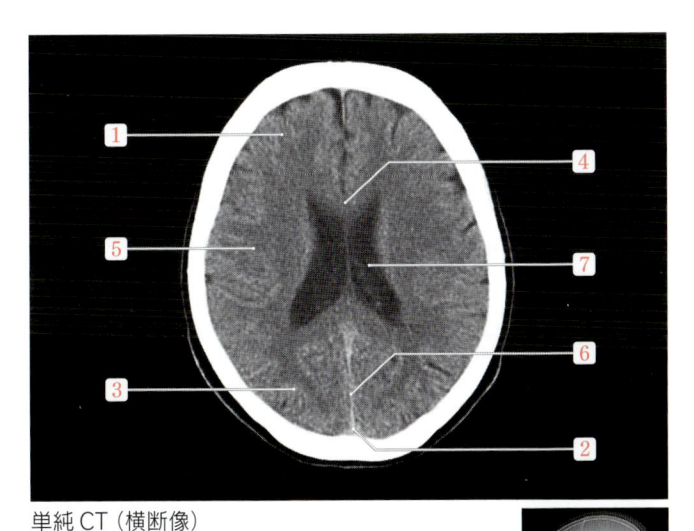

1 前頭葉　Frontal lobe
2 上矢状静脈洞　Superior sagittal sinus
3 後頭葉　Occipital lobe
4 脳梁　Corpus callosum
5 放線冠　Corona radiata
6 大脳鎌　Falx cerebri
7 側脳室　Lateral ventricle

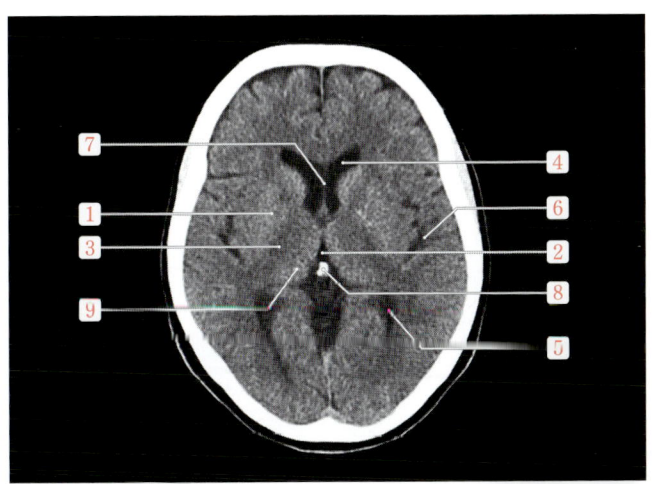

頭部

単純CT（横断像）

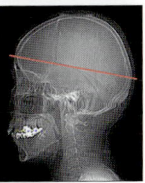

1 レンズ核　Lentiform nucleus
2 第三脳室　Third ventricle
3 内包　Internal capsule
4 側脳室前角　Anterior horn of lateral ventricle
5 側脳室後角　Posterior horn of lateral ventricle
6 Sylvius裂　Sylvian fissure
7 透明中隔　Septum pellucidum
8 松果体　Pineal body
9 視床　Thalamus

3

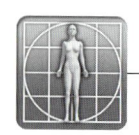

頭 部
Head

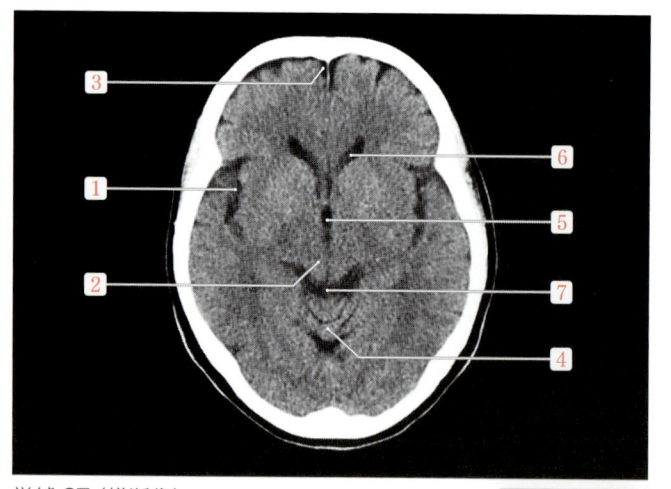

単純CT（横断像）

1 Sylvius裂　Sylvian fissure
2 中脳　Mesencephalon
3 大脳縦裂　Longitudinal fissure
4 小脳虫部　Cerebellar vermis
5 第三脳室　Third ventricle
6 側脳室前角　Anterior horn of lateral ventricle
7 四丘体槽　Quadrigeminal cistern

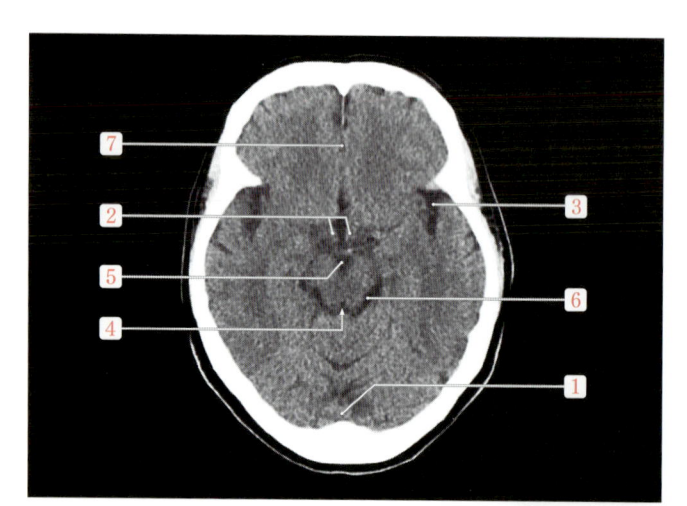

単純CT（横断像）

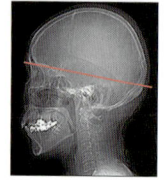

1 静脈洞交会　Sinus confluence
2 視交叉　Optic chiasm
3 Sylvius裂　Sylvian fissure
4 中脳水道　Aqueduct
5 脚間槽　Interpeduncular cistern
6 四丘体槽　Quadrigeminal cistern
7 大脳縦裂　Longitudinal fissure

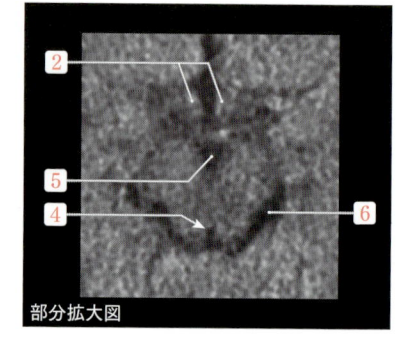

部分拡大図

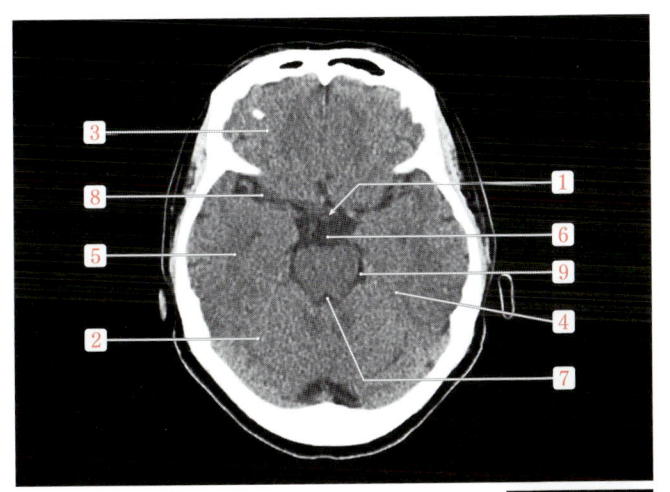

単純CT（横断像）

1 下垂体柄　Pituitary stalk
2 後頭葉　Occipital lobe
3 前頭葉　Frontal lobe
4 小脳テント　Cerebellar tentorium
5 側頭葉　Temporal lobe
6 鞍上槽　Suprasellar cistern
7 中脳水道　Aqueduct
8 Sylvius裂　Sylvian fissure
9 迂回槽　Ambient cistern

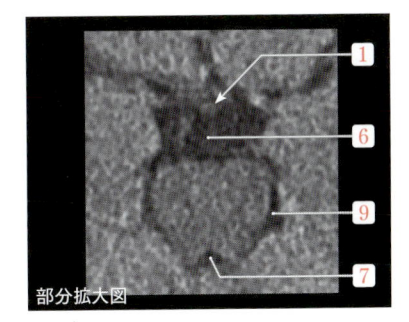

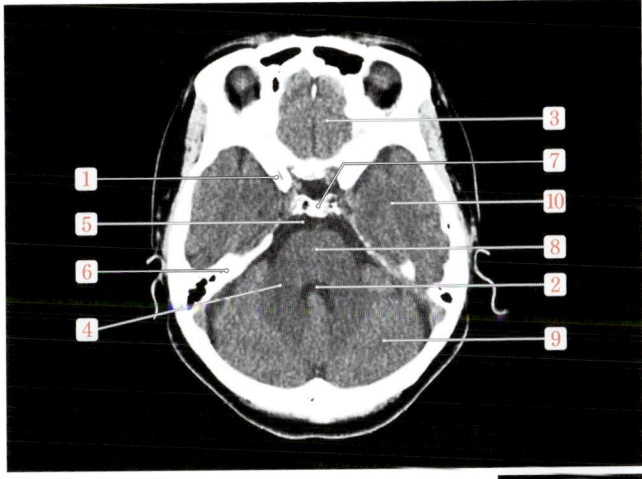

部分拡大図

単純CT（横断像）

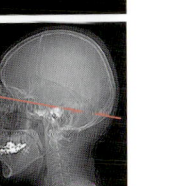

1 前床突起　Anterior clinoid process
2 第四脳室　Fourth ventricle
3 前頭葉　Frontal lobe
4 小脳脚　Cerebellar peduncle
5 橋前槽　Prepontine cistern
6 側頭骨　Temporal bone
7 トルコ鞍　Sella turcica
8 橋　Pons
9 小脳半球　Cerebellar hemisphere
10 側頭葉　Temporal lobe

頭部

頭部
Head

1 眼窩　Orbit
2 小脳半球　Cerebellar hemisphere
3 側頭葉　Temporal lobe
4 小脳橋角槽　Cerebellopontine angle cistern
5 鞍背　Dorsum sellae
6 側頭骨　Temporal bone
7 延髄　Medulla oblongata

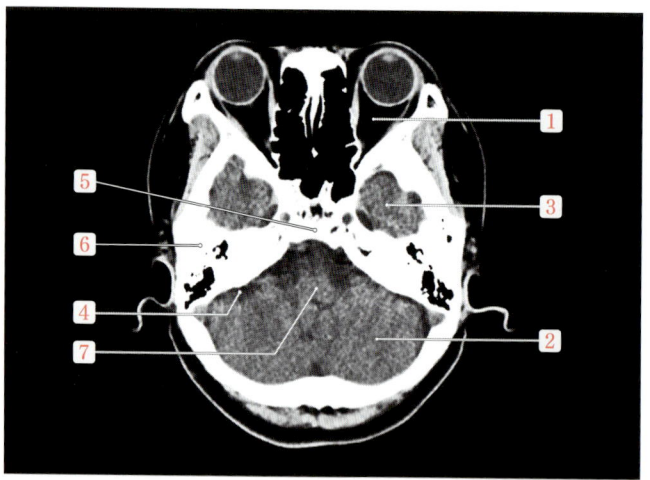

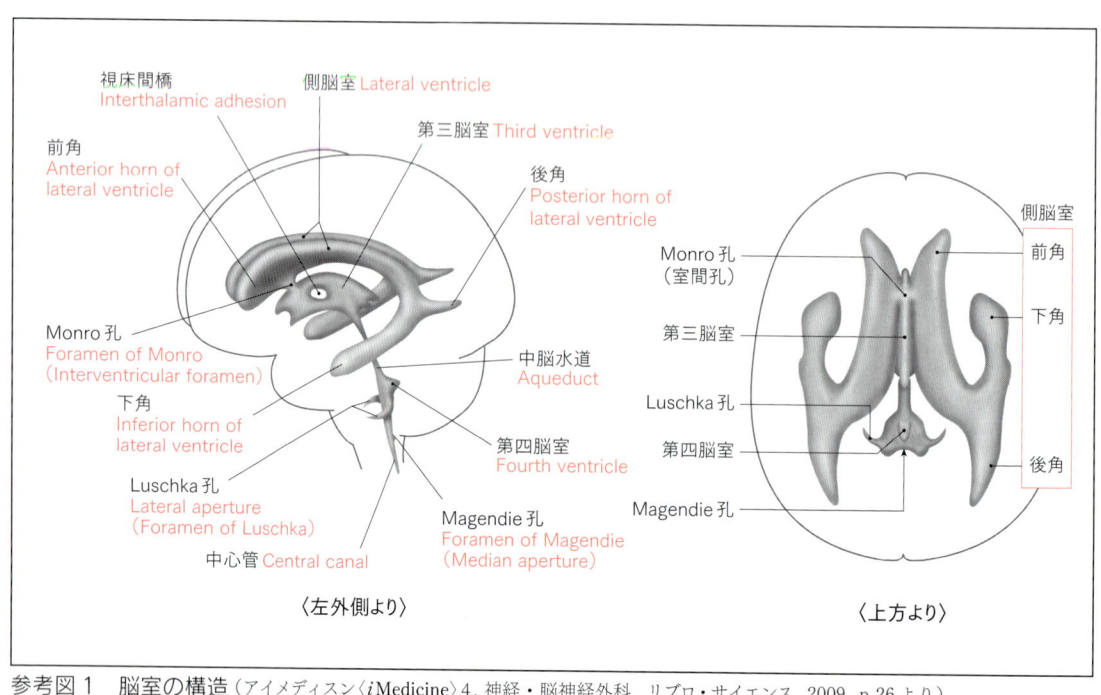

単純CT（横断像）

参考図1　脳室の構造（アイメディスン〈*i*Medicine〉4. 神経・脳神経外科. リブロ・サイエンス, 2009, p.26 より）

左外側より

- 視床間橋　Interthalamic adhesion
- 側脳室　Lateral ventricle
- 第三脳室　Third ventricle
- 前角　Anterior horn of lateral ventricle
- 後角　Posterior horn of lateral ventricle
- Monro孔　Foramen of Monro (Interventricular foramen)
- 中脳水道　Aqueduct
- 下角　Inferior horn of lateral ventricle
- 第四脳室　Fourth ventricle
- Luschka孔　Lateral aperture (Foramen of Luschka)
- 中心管　Central canal
- Magendie孔　Foramen of Magendie (Median aperture)

上方より

- 側脳室：前角／下角／後角
- Monro孔（室間孔）
- 第三脳室
- Luschka孔
- 第四脳室
- Magendie孔

6

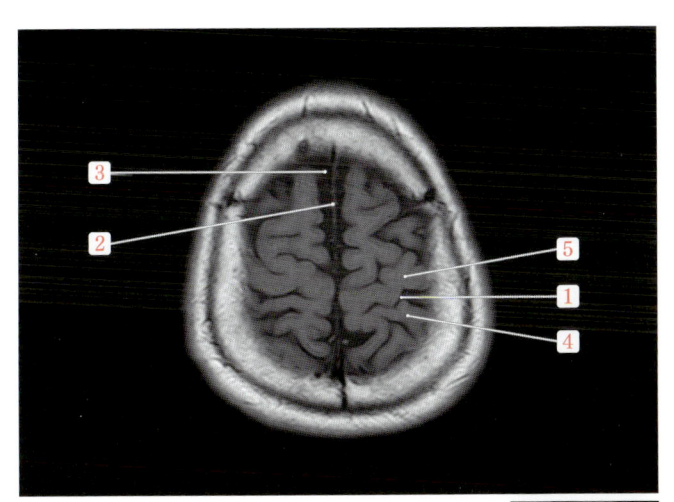

● CT・MRI 解体新書

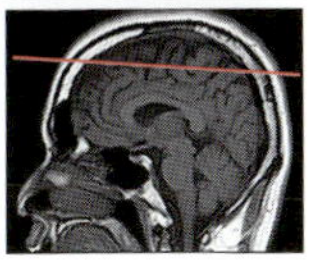

1　中心溝　　Central sulcus
2　大脳鎌　　Falx cerebri
3　大脳縦裂　Longitudinal fissure
4　中心後回　Postcentral gyrus
5　中心前回　Precentral gyrus

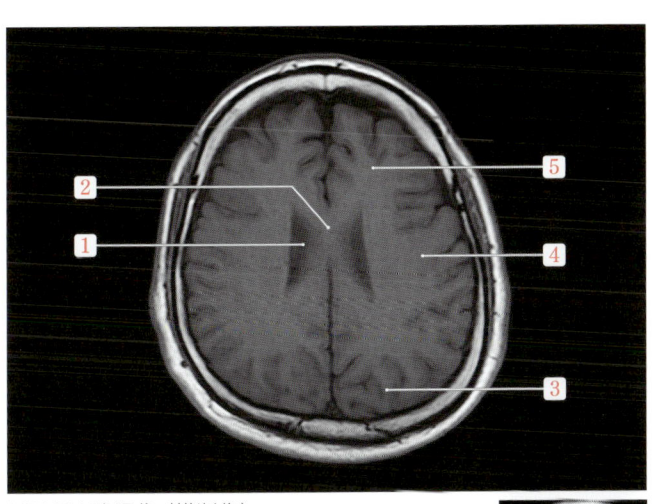

頭部

MRI T1強調像（横断像）

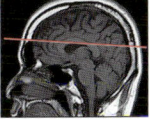

1　側脳室　Lateral ventricle
2　脳梁　　Corpus callosum
3　後頭葉　Occipital lobe
4　側頭葉　Temporal lobe
5　前頭葉　Frontal lobe

MRI T1強調像（横断像）

頭 部
Head

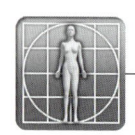

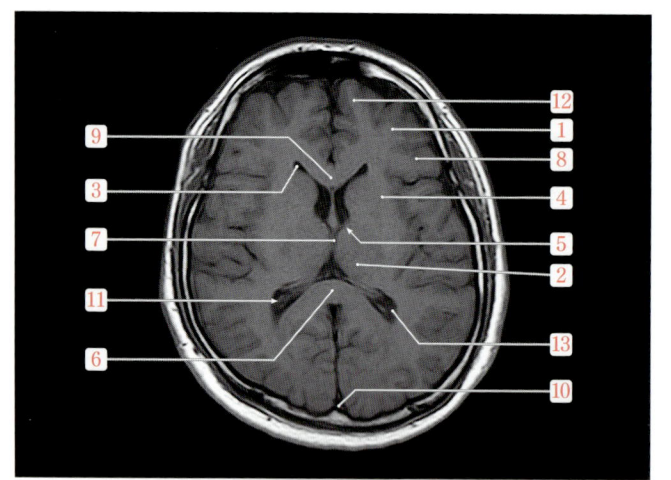

MRI T1 強調像（横断像）

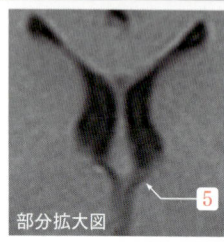

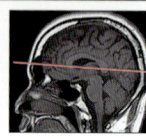

部分拡大図

1 中前頭回　Middle frontal gyrus
2 視床　Thalamus
3 側脳室前角　Anterior horn of lateral ventricle
4 レンズ核　Lentiform nucleus
5 Monro孔　Foramen of Monro
6 脳梁膨大部　Splenium of corpus callosum
7 第三脳室　Third ventricle
8 下前頭回　Inferior frontal gyrus
9 脳梁　Corpus callosum
10 上矢状静脈洞　Superior sagittal sinus
11 脈絡叢　Choroid plexus
12 上前頭回　Superior frontal gyrus
13 側脳室三角部　Trigone of lateral ventricle

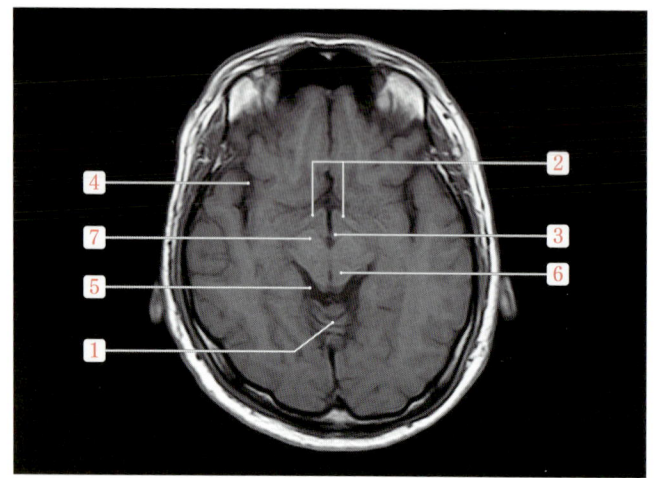

MRI T1 強調像（横断像）

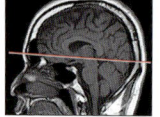

部分拡大図

1 小脳虫部　Cerebellar vermis
2 視交叉　Optic chiasm
3 乳頭体　Mammillary body
4 Sylvius裂　Sylvian fissure
5 四丘体槽　Quadrigeminal cistern
6 中脳　Mesencephalon
7 大脳脚　Cerebral peduncle

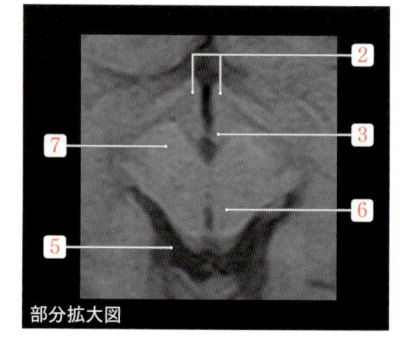

MRI T1強調像（横断像）

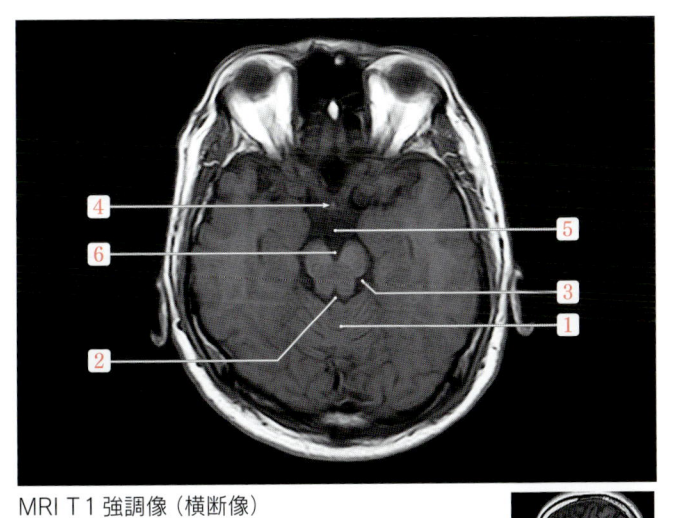

1 小脳虫部　Cerebellar vermis
2 中脳水道　Aqueduct
3 迂回槽　Ambient cistern
4 下垂体柄　Pituitary stalk
5 鞍上槽　Suprasellar cistern
6 脚間槽　Interpeduncular cistern

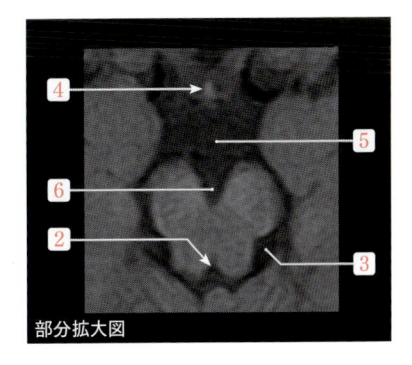

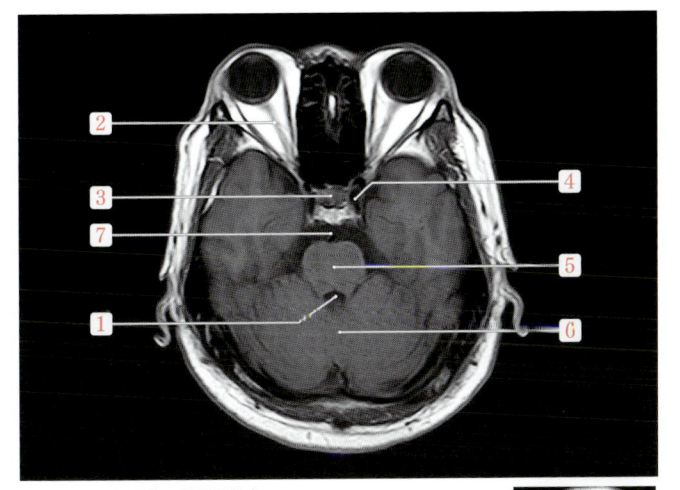

部分拡大図

MRI T1強調像（横断像）

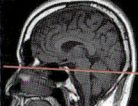

1 第四脳室　Fourth ventricle
2 視神経　Optic nerve
3 下垂体　Pituitary gland
4 内頸動脈　Internal carotid artery
5 橋　Pons
6 小脳虫部　Cerebellar vermis
7 橋前槽　Prepontine cistern

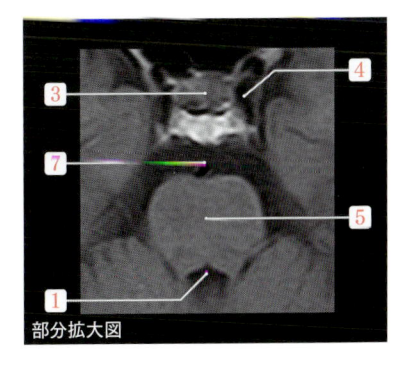

部分拡大図

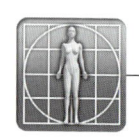

頭 部
Head

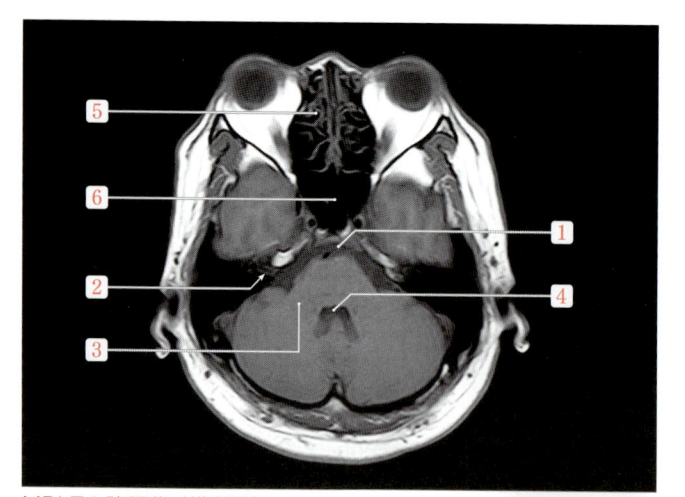

MRI T1強調像（横断像）

1 橋前槽　Prepontine cistern
2 内耳道　Internal auditory canal
3 小脳脚　Cerebellar peduncle
4 第四脳室　Fourth ventricle
5 篩骨洞　Ethmoidal sinus
6 蝶形骨洞　Sphenoidal sinus

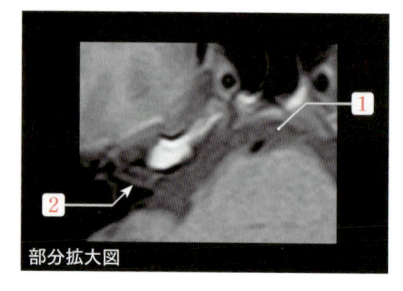

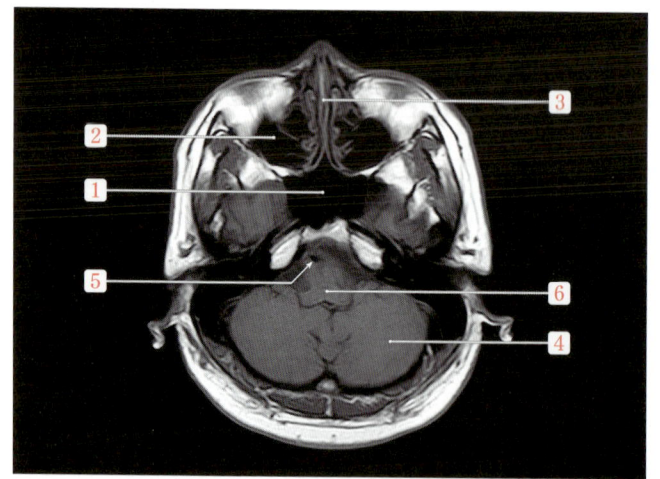

部分拡大図

MRI T1強調像（横断像）

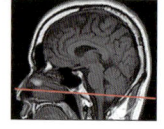

1 蝶形骨洞　Sphenoidal sinus
2 上顎洞　Maxillary sinus
3 鼻中隔　Nasal septum
4 小脳半球　Cerebellar hemisphere
5 脳底動脈　Basilar artery
6 延髄　Medulla oblongata

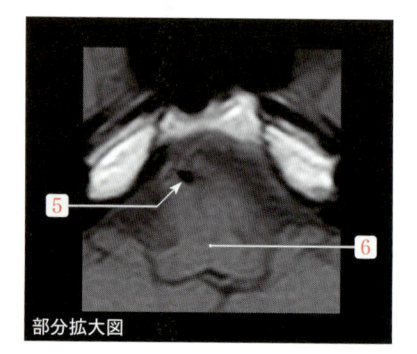

部分拡大図

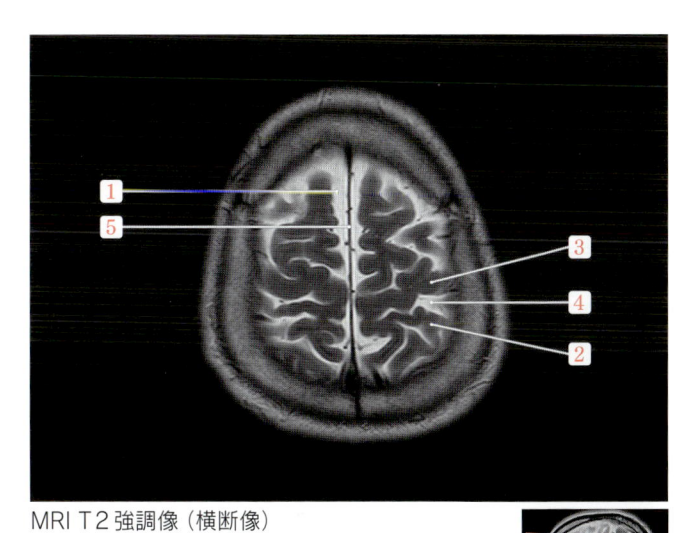

1 大脳縦裂　Longitudinal fissure
2 中心後回　Postcentral gyrus
3 中心前回　Precentral gyrus
4 中心溝　Central sulcus
5 大脳鎌　Falx cerebri

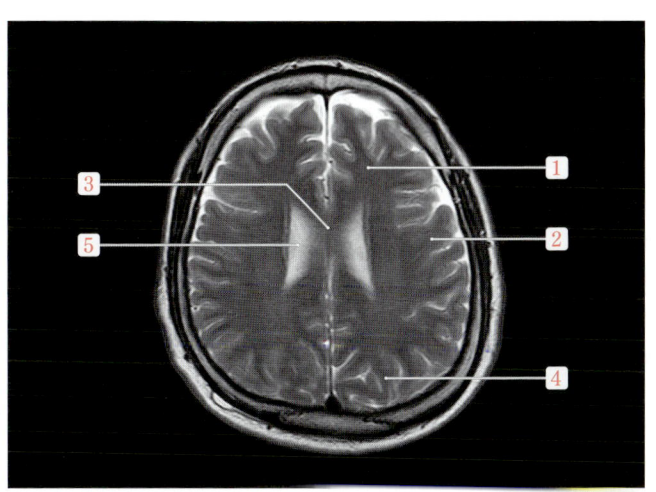

MRI T2強調像（横断像）

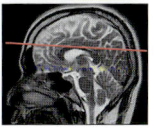

1 前頭葉　Frontal lobe
2 側頭葉　Temporal lobe
3 脳梁　Corpus callosum
4 後頭葉　Occipital lobe
5 側脳室　Lateral ventricle

MRI T2強調像（横断像）

頭 部
Head

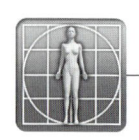

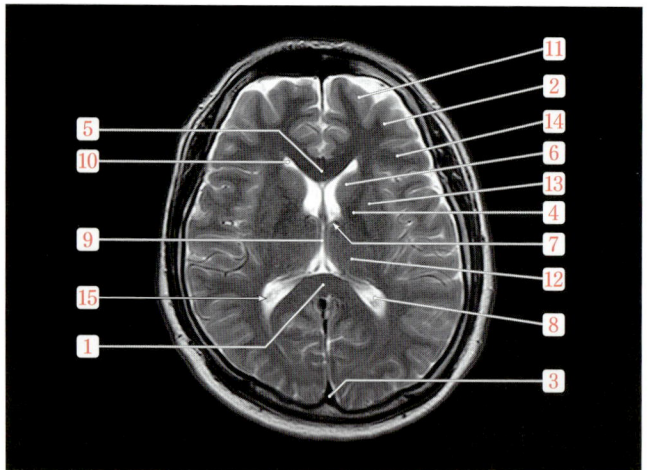

MRI T2強調像（横断像）

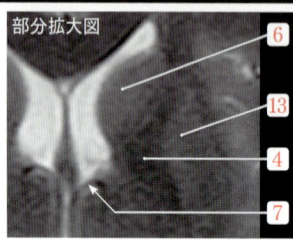

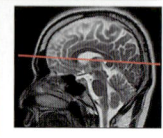

部分拡大図

1 脳梁膨大部　Splenium of corpus callosum
2 中前頭回　Middle frontal gyrus
3 上矢状静脈洞　Superior sagittal sinus
4 内包　Internal capsule
5 脳梁　Corpus callosum
6 尾状核　Caudate nucleus
7 Monro孔　Foramen of Monro
8 側脳室三角部　Trigone of lateral ventricle
9 第三脳室　Third ventricle
10 側脳室前角　Anterior horn of lateral ventricle
11 上前頭回　Superior frontal gyrus
12 視床　Thalamus
13 レンズ核　Lentiform nucleus
14 下前頭回　Inferior frontal gyrus
15 脈絡叢　Choroid plexus

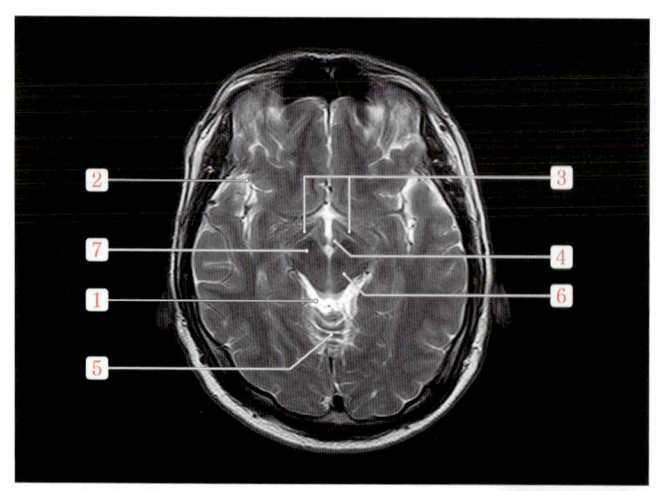

MRI T2強調像（横断像）

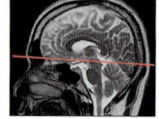

1 四丘体槽　Quadrigeminal cistern
2 Sylvius裂　Sylvian fissure
3 視交叉　Optic chiasm
4 乳頭体　Mammillary body
5 小脳虫部　Cerebellar vermis
6 中脳　Mesencephalon
7 大脳脚　Cerebral peduncle

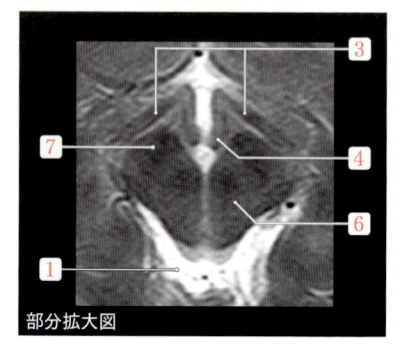

部分拡大図

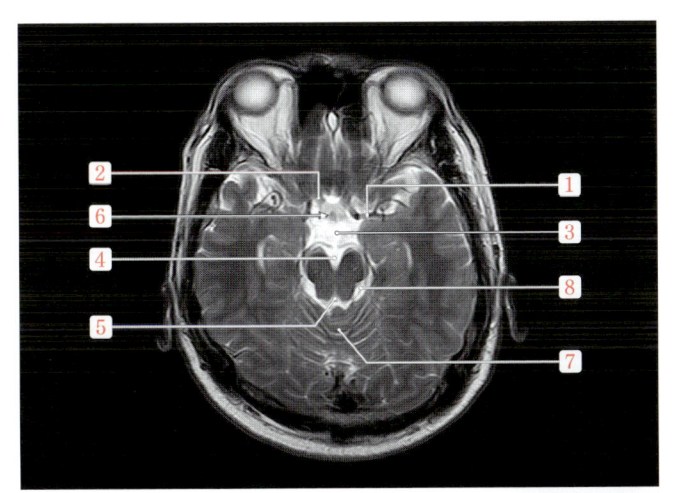

1 中大脳動脈　Middle cerebral artery
2 右視神経　Right optic nerve
3 鞍上槽　Suprasellar cistern
4 脚間槽　Interpeduncular cistern
5 中脳水道　Aqueduct
6 下垂体柄　Pituitary stalk
7 小脳虫部　Cerebellar vermis
8 迂回槽　Ambient cistern

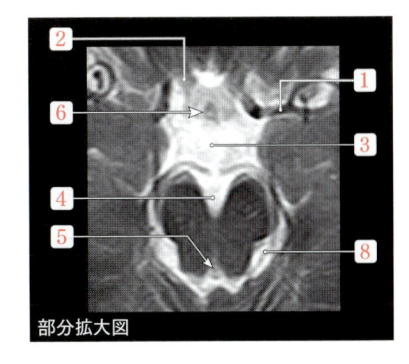

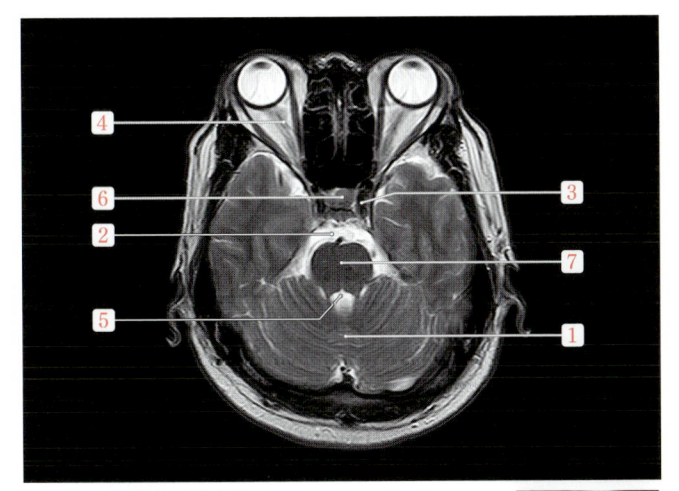

MRI T2強調像（横断像）

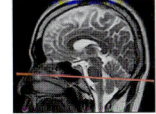

部分拡大図

1 小脳虫部　Cerebellar vermis
2 橋前槽　Prepontine cistern
3 内頸動脈　Internal carotid artery
4 視神経　Optic nerve
5 第四脳室　Fourth ventricle
6 下垂体　Pituitary gland
7 橋　Pons

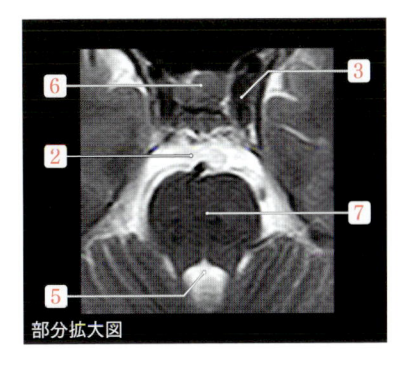

MRI T2強調像（横断像）

部分拡大図

CT・MRI解体新書

頭部

13

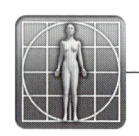

頭 部
Head

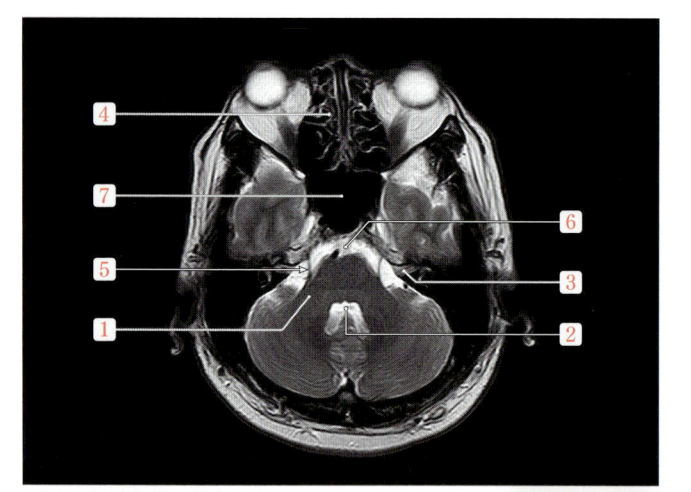

MRI T2強調像（横断像）

1 小脳脚　Cerebellar peduncle
2 第四脳室　Fourth ventricle
3 内耳道　Internal auditory canal
4 篩骨洞　Ethmoidal sinus
5 三叉神経　Trigeminal nerve
6 橋前槽　Prepontine cistern
7 蝶形骨洞　Sphenoidal sinus

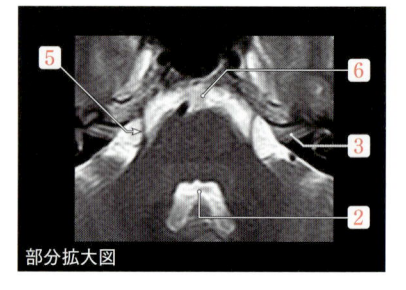

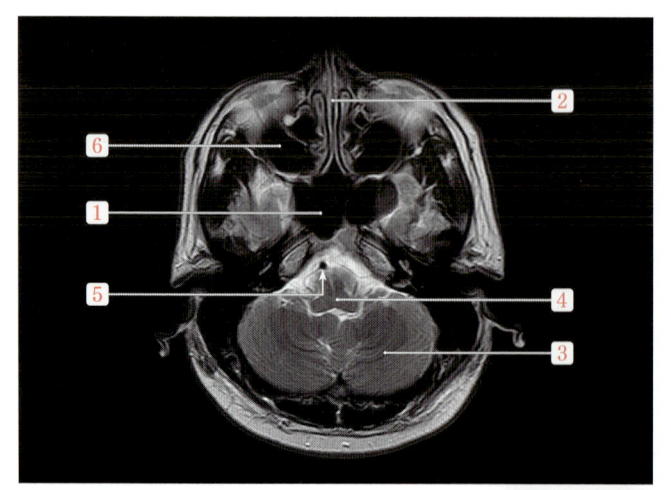

部分拡大図

MRI T2強調像（横断像）

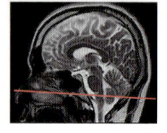

1 蝶形骨洞　Sphenoidal sinus
2 鼻中隔　Nasal septum
3 小脳半球　Cerebellar hemisphere
4 延髄　Medulla oblongata
5 脳底動脈　Basilar artery
6 上顎洞　Maxillary sinus

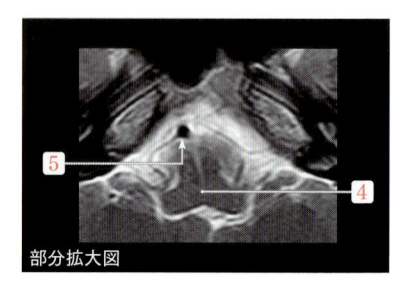

部分拡大図

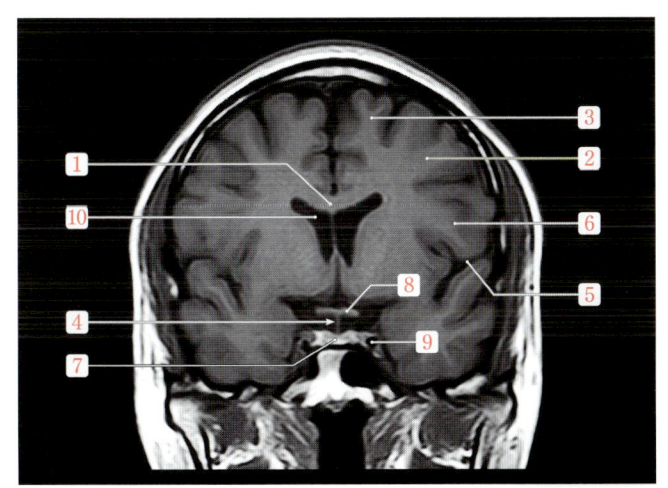

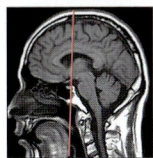

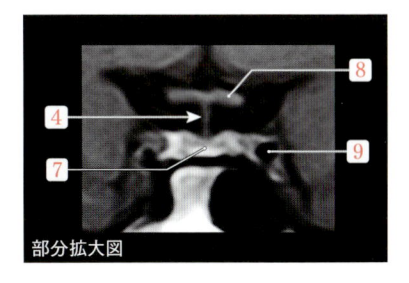

1 脳梁　Corpus callosum
2 中前頭回　Middle frontal gyrus
3 上前頭回　Superior frontal gyrus
4 下垂体柄　Pituitary stalk
5 Sylvius裂　Sylvian fissure
6 下前頭回　Inferior frontal gyrus
7 下垂体　Pituitary gland
8 視交叉　Optic chiasm
9 内頸動脈　Internal carotid artery
10 側脳室　Lateral ventricle

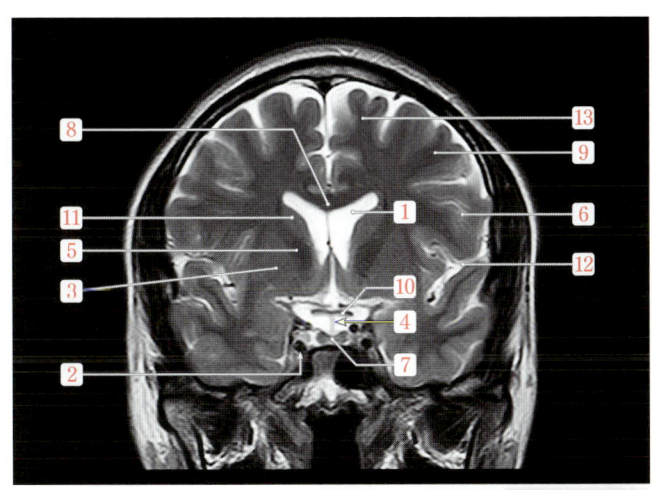

MRI T1強調像（冠状断像）

部分拡大図

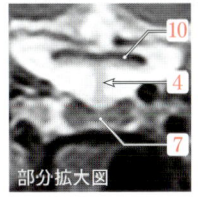

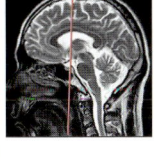

1 側脳室　Lateral ventricle
2 内頸動脈　Internal carotid artery
3 レンズ核　Lentiform nucleus
4 下垂体柄　Pituitary stalk
5 内包　Internal capsule
6 下前頭回　Inferior frontal gyrus
7 下垂体　Pituitary gland
8 脳梁　Corpus callosum
9 中前頭回　Middle frontal gyrus
10 視交叉　Optic chiasm
11 尾状核　Caudate nucleus
12 Sylvius裂　Sylvian fissure
13 上前頭回　Superior frontal gyrus

MRI T2強調像（冠状断像）

部分拡大図

頭部

頭部
Head

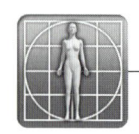

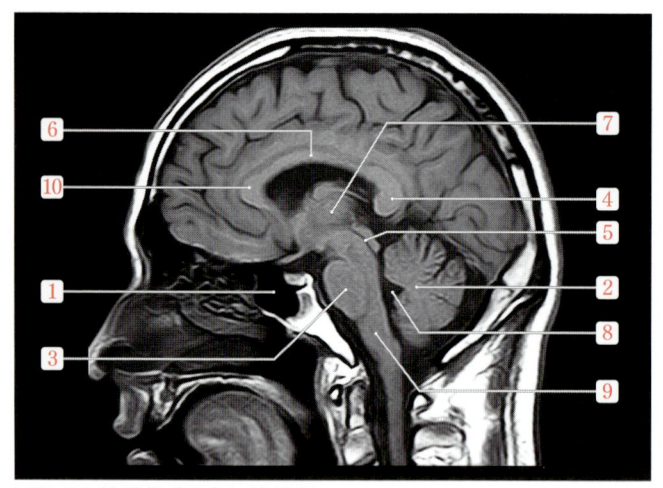

MRI T1強調像（正中矢状断像）

1 蝶形骨洞　Sphenoidal sinus
2 小脳半球　Cerebellar hemisphere
3 橋　Pons
4 脳梁膨大部　Splenium of corpus callosum
5 中脳水道　Aqueduct
6 脳梁体部　Body of corpus callosum
7 視床間橋　Interthalamic adhesion
8 第四脳室　Fourth ventricle
9 延髄　Medulla oblongata
10 脳梁膝部　Genu of corpus callosum

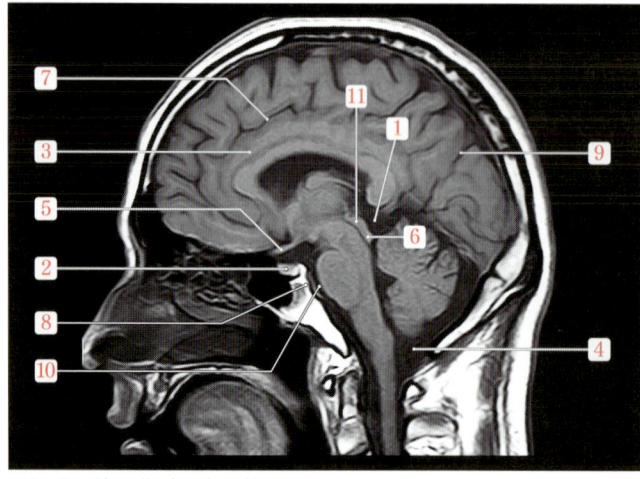

MRI T1強調像（正中矢状断像）

1 四丘体槽　Quadrigeminal cistern
2 下垂体　Pituitary gland
3 帯状回　Cingulate gyrus
4 大槽　Cisterna magna
5 視神経　Optic nerve
6 下丘　Inferior colliculus
7 帯状溝　Cingulate sulcus
8 鞍背　Dorsum sellae
9 頭頂後頭溝　Parieto-occipital sulcus
10 橋前槽　Prepontine cistern
11 上丘　Superior colliculus

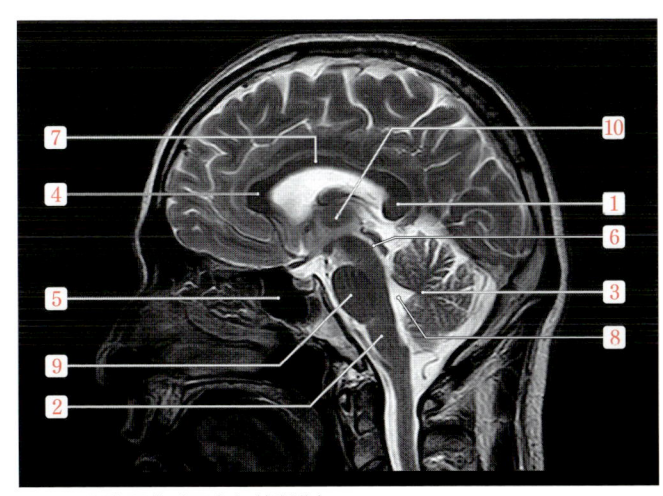

1 脳梁膨大部　Splenium of corpus callosum
2 延髄　Medulla oblongata
3 小脳半球　Cerebellar hemisphere
4 脳梁膝部　Genu of corpus callosum
5 蝶形骨洞　Sphenoidal sinus
6 中脳水道　Aqueduct
7 脳梁体部　Body of corpus callosum
8 第四脳室　Fourth ventricle
9 橋　Pons
10 視床間橋　Interthalamic adhesion

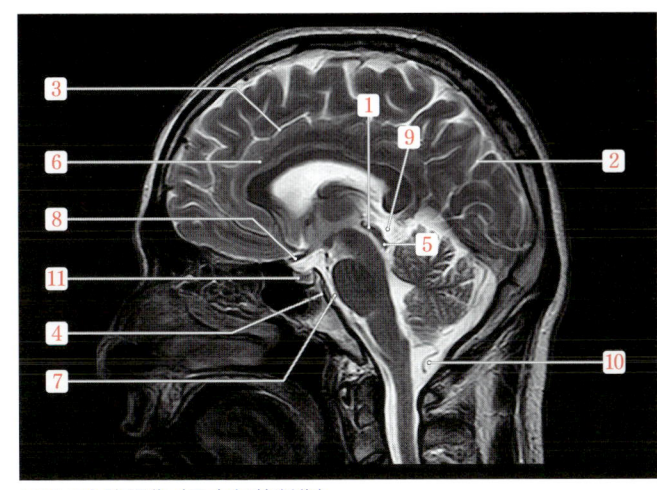

MRI T2強調像（正中矢状断像）

1 上丘　Superior colliculus
2 頭頂後頭溝　Parieto-occipital sulcus
3 帯状溝　Cingulate sulcus
4 鞍背　Dorsum sellae
5 下丘　Inferior colliculus
6 帯状回　Cingulate gyrus
7 橋前槽　Prepontine cistern
8 視神経　Optic nerve
9 四丘体槽　Quadrigeminal cistern
10 大槽　Cisterna magna
11 下垂体　Pituitary gland

MRI T2強調像（正中矢状断像）

● CT・MRI解体新書

頭部

頭 部
Head

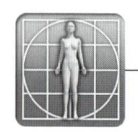

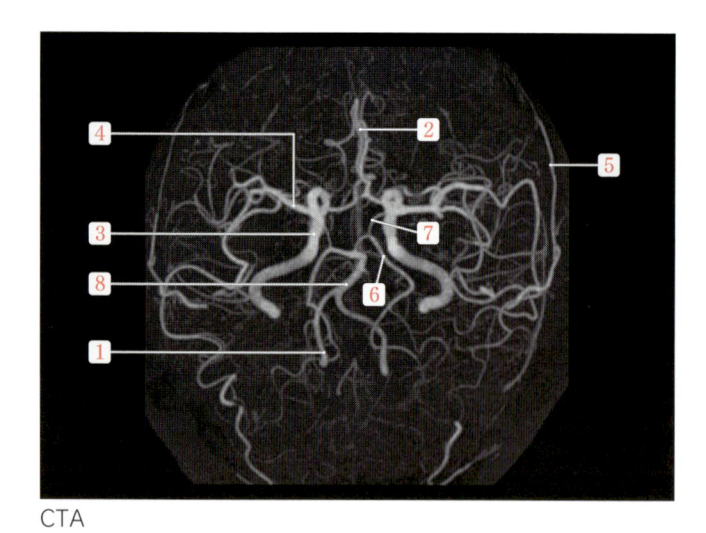

CTA

1 椎骨動脈　Vertebral artery
2 前大脳動脈　Anterior cerebral artery
3 内頸動脈　Internal carotid artery
4 中大脳動脈　Middle cerebral artery
5 浅側頭動脈　Superficial temporal artery
6 後大脳動脈　Posterior cerebral artery
7 後交通動脈
　Posterior communicating artery
8 脳底動脈　Basilar artery

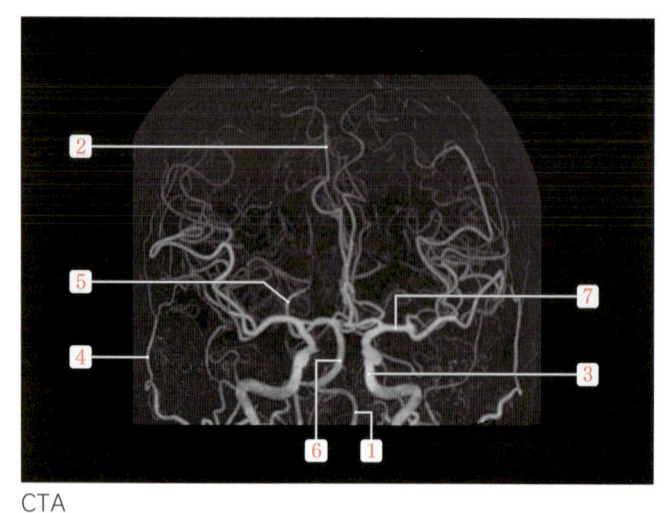

CTA

1 椎骨動脈　Vertebral artery
2 前大脳動脈　Anterior cerebral artery
3 内頸動脈　Internal carotid artery
4 浅側頭動脈　Superficial temporal artery
5 後大脳動脈　Posterior cerebral artery
6 脳底動脈　Basilar artery
7 中大脳動脈　Middle cerebral artery

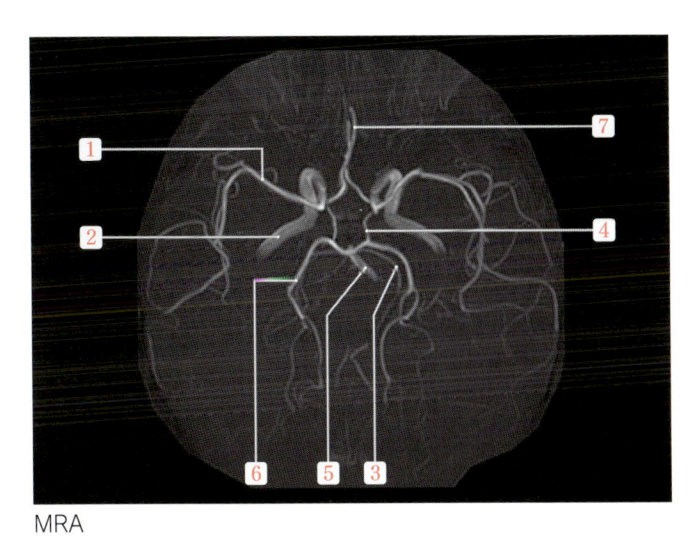

1 中大脳動脈　Middle cerebral artery
2 内頸動脈　Internal carotid artery
3 上小脳動脈　Superior cerebellar artery
4 後交通動脈
　Posterior communicating artery
5 脳底動脈　Basilar artery
6 後大脳動脈　Posterior cerebral artery
7 前大脳動脈　Anterior cerebral artery

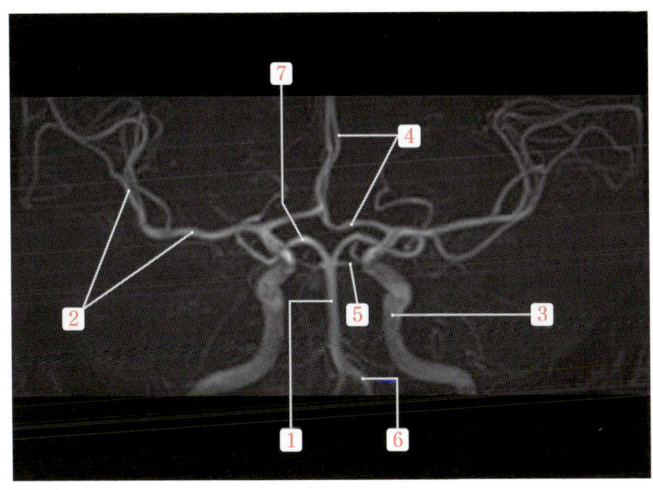

MRA

1 脳底動脈　Basilar artery
2 中大脳動脈　Middle cerebral artery
3 内頸動脈　Internal carotid artery
4 前大脳動脈　Anterior cerebral artery
5 上小脳動脈　Superior cerebellar artery
6 椎骨動脈　Vertebral artery
7 後大脳動脈　Posterior cerebral artery

MRA

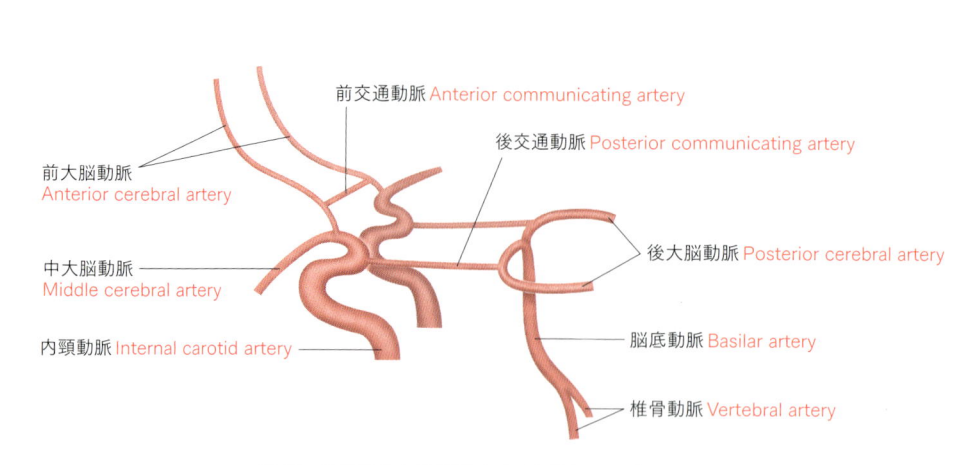

頭部
Head

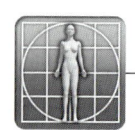

〈Willis動脈輪を左外側後上方より見たところ〉

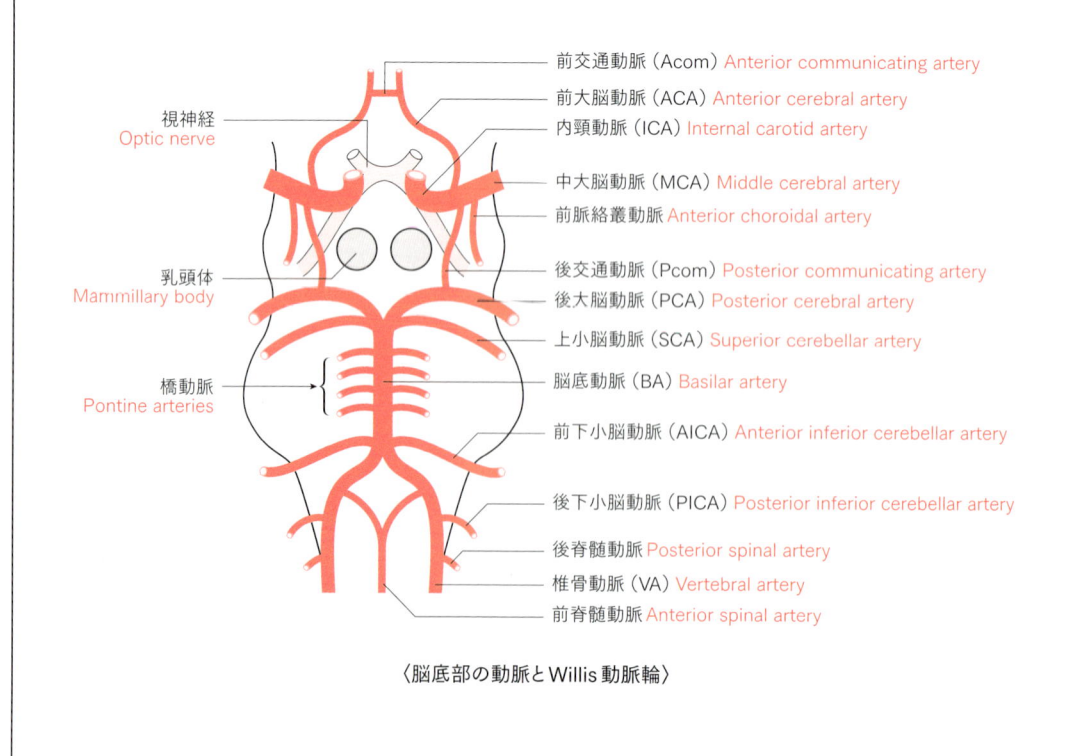

- 前交通動脈 Anterior communicating artery
- 前大脳動脈 Anterior cerebral artery
- 後交通動脈 Posterior communicating artery
- 中大脳動脈 Middle cerebral artery
- 後大脳動脈 Posterior cerebral artery
- 内頸動脈 Internal carotid artery
- 脳底動脈 Basilar artery
- 椎骨動脈 Vertebral artery

〈脳底部の動脈とWillis動脈輪〉

- 視神経 Optic nerve
- 乳頭体 Mammillary body
- 橋動脈 Pontine arteries
- 前交通動脈（Acom）Anterior communicating artery
- 前大脳動脈（ACA）Anterior cerebral artery
- 内頸動脈（ICA）Internal carotid artery
- 中大脳動脈（MCA）Middle cerebral artery
- 前脈絡叢動脈 Anterior choroidal artery
- 後交通動脈（Pcom）Posterior communicating artery
- 後大脳動脈（PCA）Posterior cerebral artery
- 上小脳動脈（SCA）Superior cerebellar artery
- 脳底動脈（BA）Basilar artery
- 前下小脳動脈（AICA）Anterior inferior cerebellar artery
- 後下小脳動脈（PICA）Posterior inferior cerebellar artery
- 後脊髄動脈 Posterior spinal artery
- 椎骨動脈（VA）Vertebral artery
- 前脊髄動脈 Anterior spinal artery

参考図2　Willis動脈輪（アイメディスン〈iMedicine〉4．神経・脳神経外科．リブロ・サイエンス，2009, p.45・49 より）

CT・MRI
解体新書
- 正常解剖 -

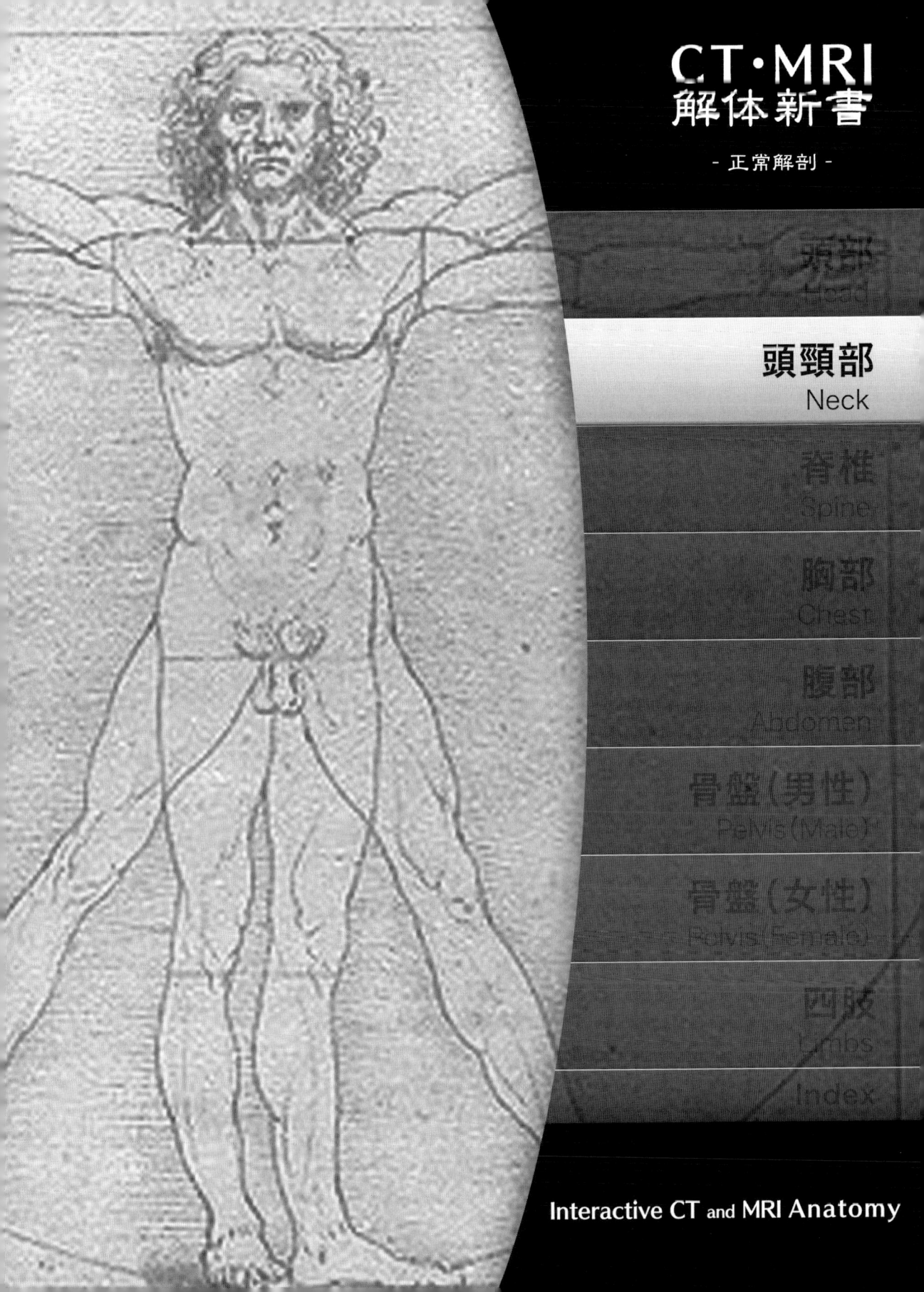

頭頸部
Neck

脊椎
Spine

胸部
Chest

腹部
Abdomen

骨盤（男性）
Pelvis (Male)

骨盤（女性）
Pelvis (Female)

四肢
Limbs

Index

Interactive CT and MRI Anatomy

頭頸部
Neck

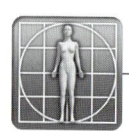

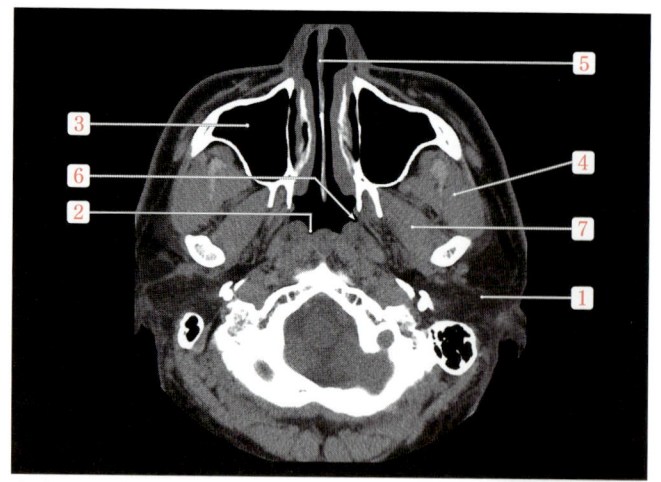

単純CT（横断像）

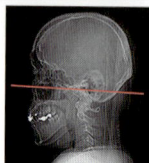

1 耳下腺　　Parotid gland
2 ローゼンミューラー窩　　Rosenmüller's fossa
3 上顎洞　　Maxillary sinus
4 咬筋　　Masseter
5 鼻中隔　　Nasal septum
6 耳管咽頭口　　Pharyngeal orifice of eustachian tube
7 外側翼突筋　　Lateral pterygoid

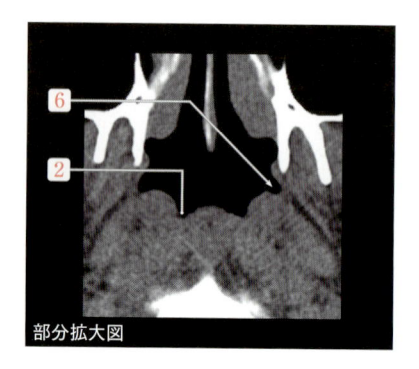

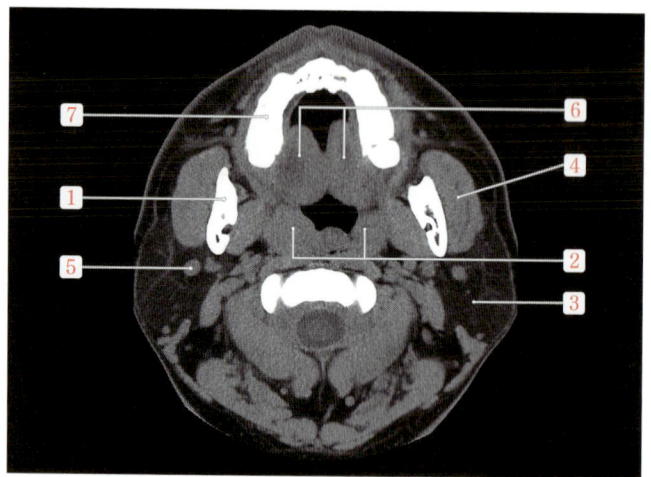

部分拡大図

単純CT（横断像）

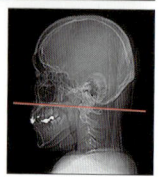

1 下顎骨下顎枝　　Ramus of mandible
2 口蓋扁桃　　Palatine tonsil
3 耳下腺　　Parotid gland
4 咬筋　　Masseter
5 下顎後静脈　　Retromandibular vein
6 舌　　Tongue
7 上顎骨　　Maxilla

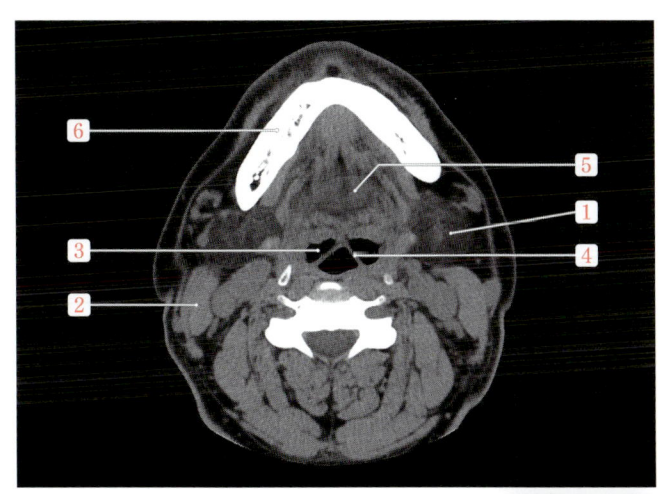

1 顎下腺　Submandibular gland
2 胸鎖乳突筋　Sternocleidomastoid
3 喉頭蓋谷　Vallecula epiglottica
4 喉頭蓋　Epiglottis
5 顎二腹筋　Digastric
6 下顎骨　Mandible

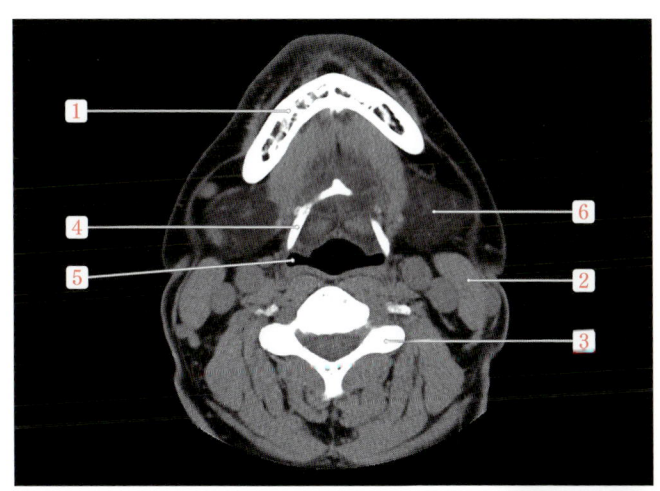

単純CT（横断像）

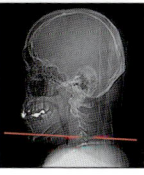

1 下顎骨　Mandible
2 胸鎖乳突筋　Sternocleidomastoid
3 頸椎　Cervical vertebra
4 舌骨　Hyoid bone
5 梨状陥凹　Piriform fossa
6 顎下腺　Submandibular gland

単純CT（横断像）

頭頸部

23

頭頸部
Neck

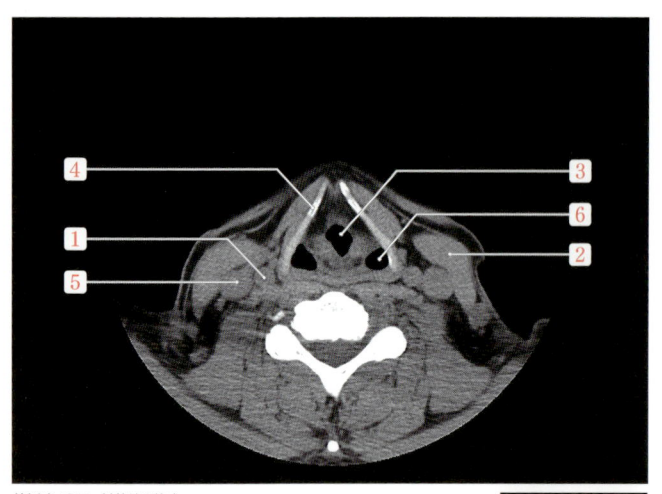

1 総頸動脈　Common carotid artery
2 胸鎖乳突筋　Sternocleidomastoid
3 喉頭　Larynx
4 甲状軟骨　Thyroid cartilage
5 内頸静脈　Internal jugular vein
6 梨状陥凹　Piriform fossa

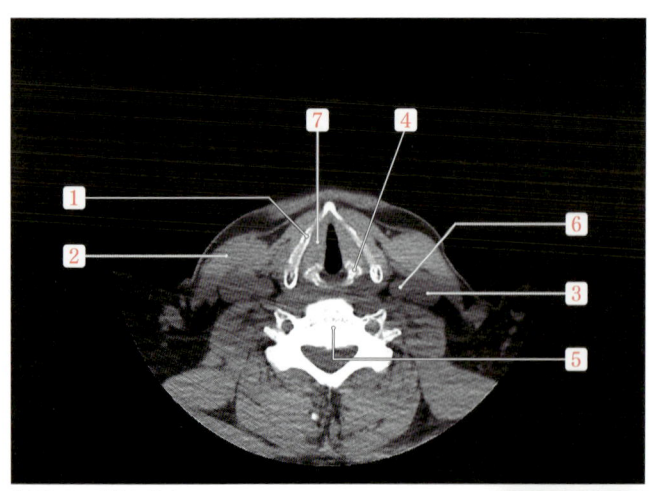

単純CT（横断像）

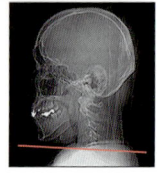

1 甲状軟骨　Thyroid cartilage
2 胸鎖乳突筋　Sternocleidomastoid
3 内頸静脈　Internal jugular vein
4 披裂軟骨　Arytenoid cartilage
5 頸椎　Cervical vertebral body
6 総頸動脈　Common carotid artery
7 声帯　Vocal cord

単純CT（横断像）

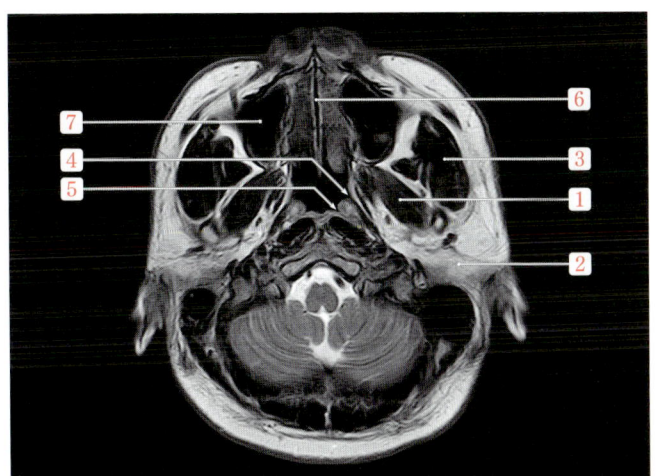

MRI T2強調像（横断像）

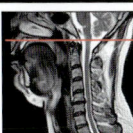

1 外側翼突筋　Lateral pterygoid
2 耳下腺　Parotid gland
3 咬筋　Masseter
4 耳管咽頭口　Pharyngeal orifice of eustachian tube
5 ローゼンミューフー窩　Rosenmüller's fossa
6 鼻中隔　Nasal septum
7 上顎洞　Maxillary sinus

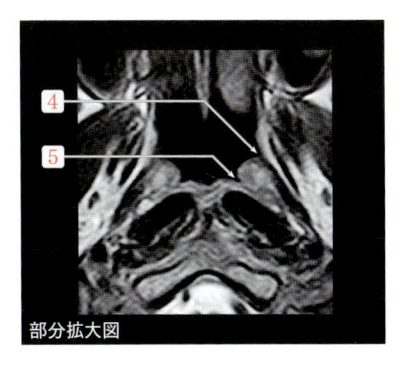

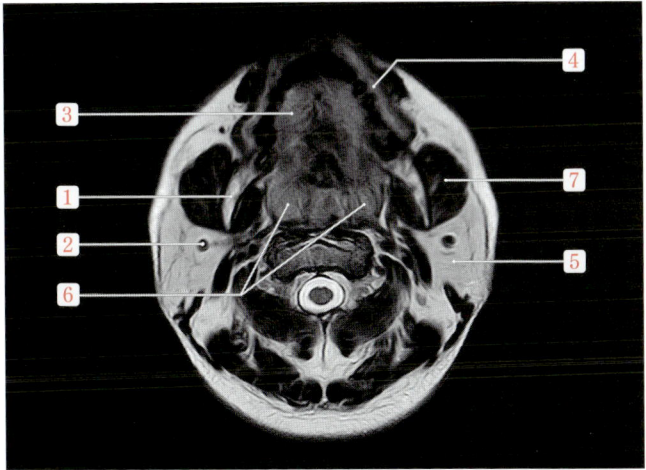

部分拡大図

MRI T2強調像（横断像）

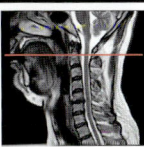

1 下顎骨下顎枝　Ramus of mandible
2 下顎後静脈　Retromandibular vein
3 舌　Tongue
4 上顎骨　Maxilla
5 耳下腺　Parotid gland
6 口蓋扁桃　Palatine tonsil
7 咬筋　Masseter

頭頸部
Neck

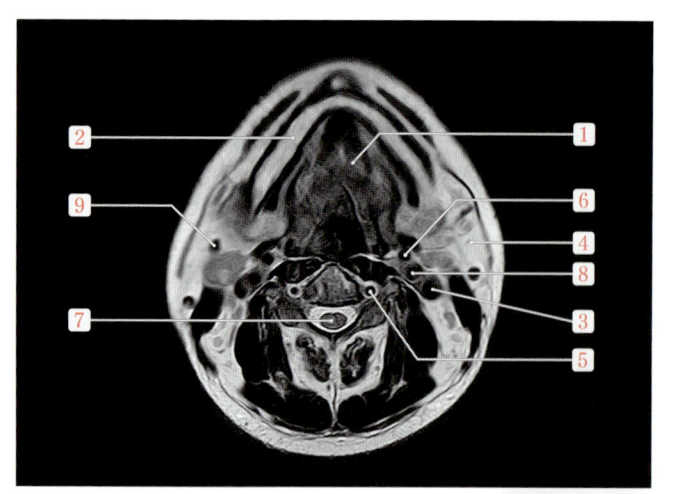

MRI T2 強調像（横断像）

1 顎二腹筋　Digastric
2 下顎骨　Mandible
3 内頸静脈　Internal jugular vein
4 顎下腺　Submandibular gland
5 椎骨動脈　Vertebral artery
6 外頸動脈　External carotid artery
7 頸髄　Cervical spinal cord
8 内頸動脈　Internal carotid artery
9 下顎後静脈　Retromandibular vein

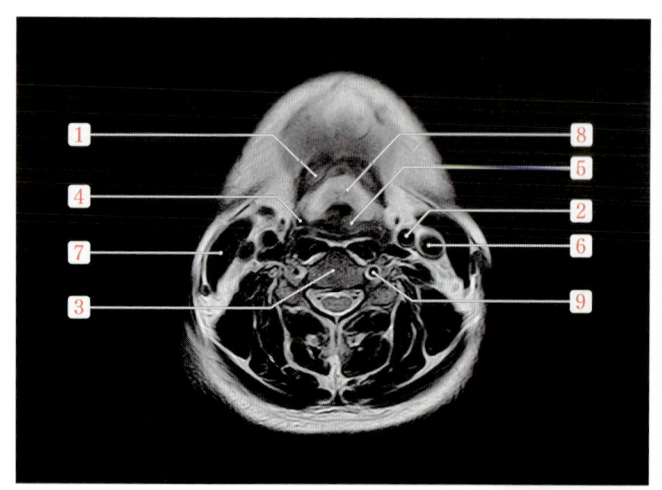

MRI T2 強調像（横断像）

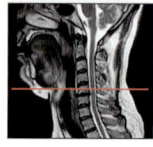

1 舌骨　Hyoid bone
2 総頸動脈　Common carotid artery
3 頸椎椎体　Cervical vertebral body
4 梨状陥凹　Piriform fossa
5 披裂喉頭蓋ヒダ　Ary-epiglottic fold
6 内頸静脈　Internal jugular vein
7 胸鎖乳突筋　Sternocleidomastoid
8 前喉頭蓋間隙　Pre-epiglottic space
9 椎骨動脈　Vertebral artery

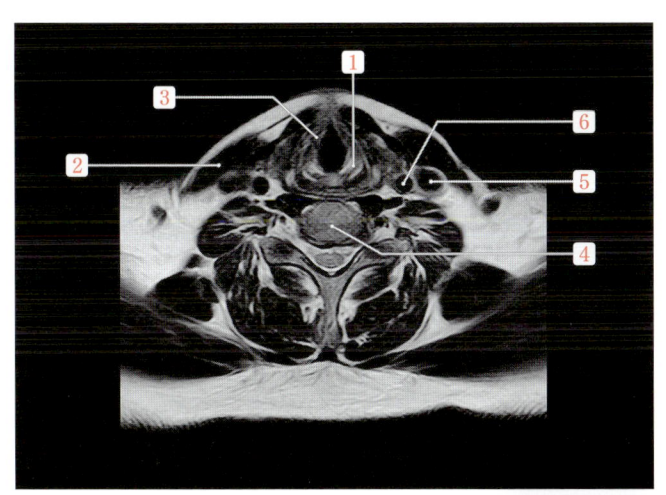

MRI T2強調像（横断像）

1 披裂軟骨　Arytenoid cartilage
2 胸鎖乳突筋　Sternocleidomastoid
3 声帯　Vocal cord
4 頸椎椎体　Cervical vertebral body
5 内頸静脈　Internal jugular vein
6 総頸動脈　Common carotid artery

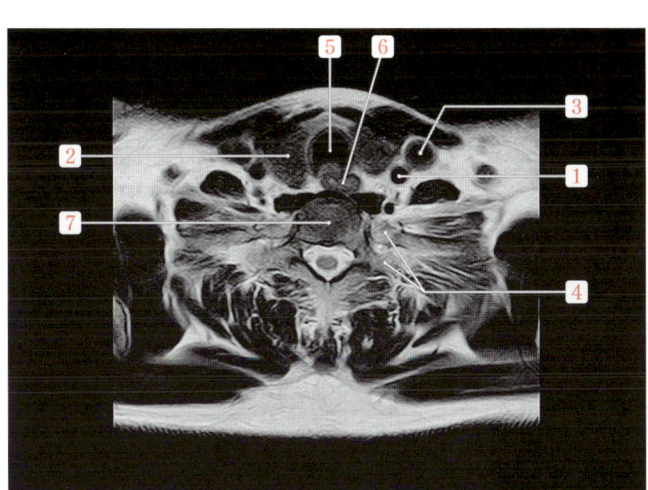

MRI T2強調像（横断像）

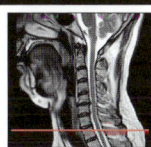

1 総頸動脈　Common carotid artery
2 甲状腺　Thyroid gland
3 内頸静脈　Internal jugular vein
4 肋骨　Ribs
5 気管　Trachea
6 食道　Esophagus
7 胸椎　Thoracic vertebra

頭頸部
Neck

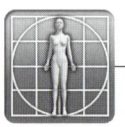

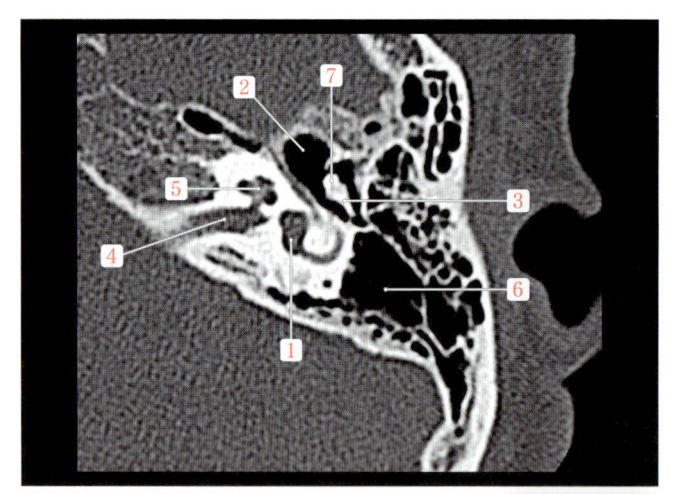

高分解能 CT（横断像）

1 外側半規管　Lateral semicircular canal
2 前鼓室上陥凹　Anterior epitympanic recess
3 アブミ骨　Stapes
4 内耳道　Internal auditory canal
5 蝸牛　Cochlea
6 乳突洞　Mastoid antrum
7 ツチ骨　Malleus

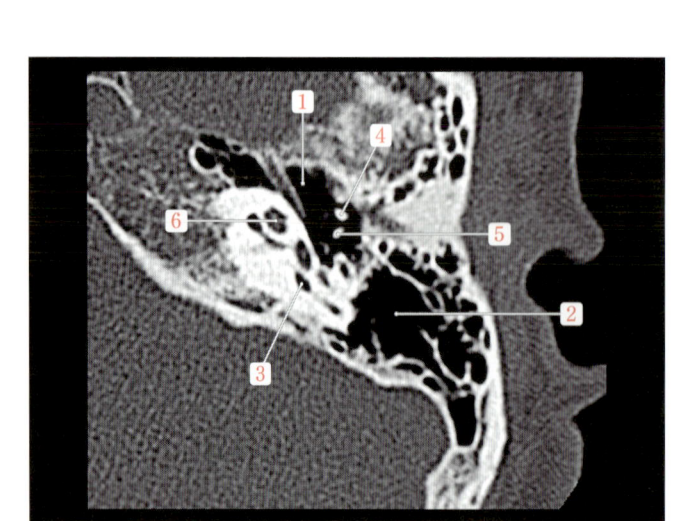

高分解能 CT（横断像）

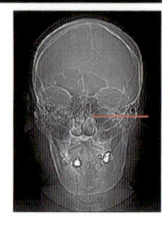

1 前鼓室上陥凹　Anterior epitympanic recess
2 乳突洞　Mastoid antrum
3 後半規管　Posterior semicircular canal
4 ツチ骨　Malleus
5 キヌタ骨　Incus
6 蝸牛　Cochlea

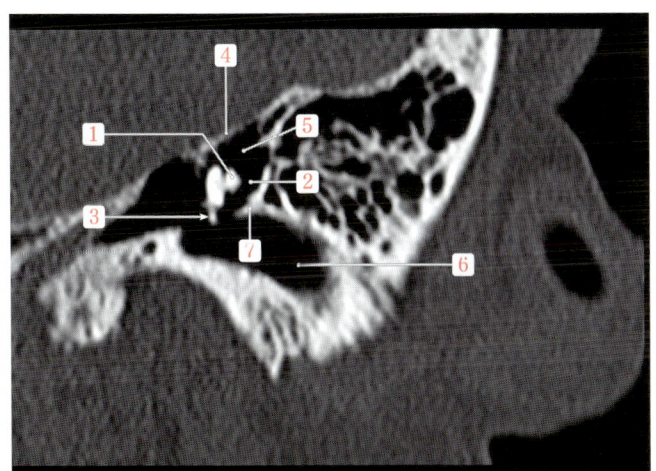

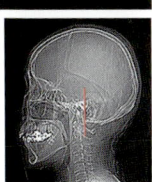

1 ツチ骨　Malleus
2 プルサック腔　Prussak's space
3 アブミ骨　Stapes
4 鼓室蓋　Tegmen tympani
5 鼓室上陥凹　Epitympanic recess
6 外耳道　External auditory canal
7 鼓膜被蓋　Scutum

高分解能CT（冠状断像）

頭頸部
Neck

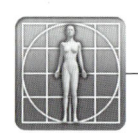

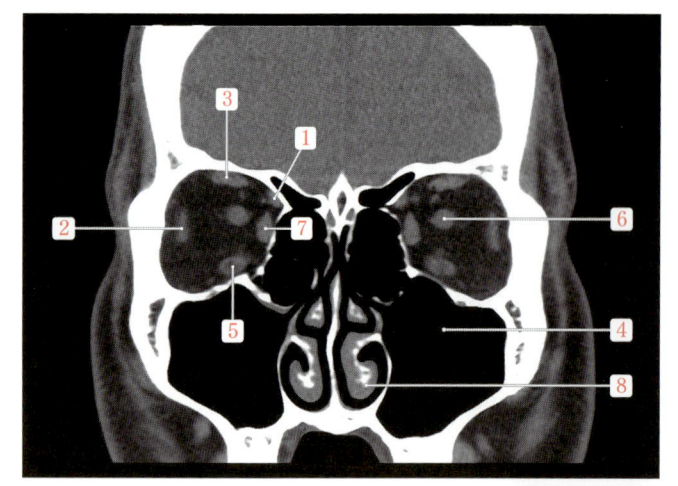

単純 CT（冠状断像）

1 上斜筋　Superior oblique
2 外側直筋　Lateral rectus
3 上直筋　Superior rectus
4 上顎洞　Maxillary sinus
5 下直筋　Inferior rectus
6 視神経　Optic nerve
7 内側直筋　Medial rectus
8 下鼻甲介　Inferior nasal concha

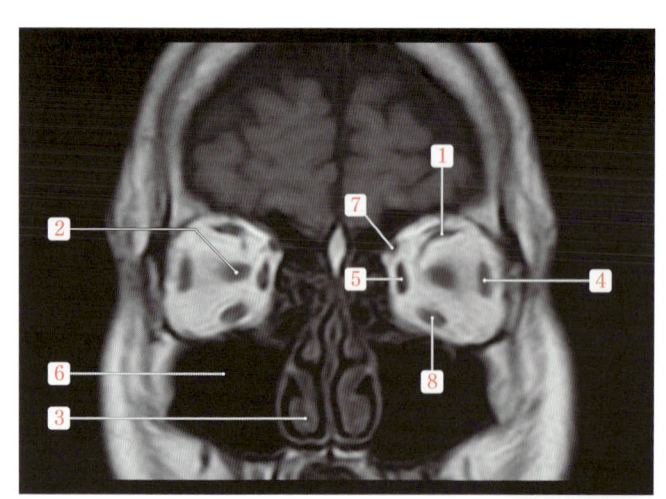

MRI T1 強調像（冠状断像）

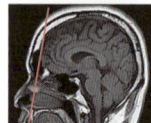

1 上直筋　Superior rectus
2 視神経　Optic nerve
3 下鼻甲介　Inferior nasal concha
4 外側直筋　Lateral rectus
5 内側直筋　Medial rectus
6 上顎洞　Maxillary sinus
7 上斜筋　Superior oblique
8 下直筋　Inferior rectus

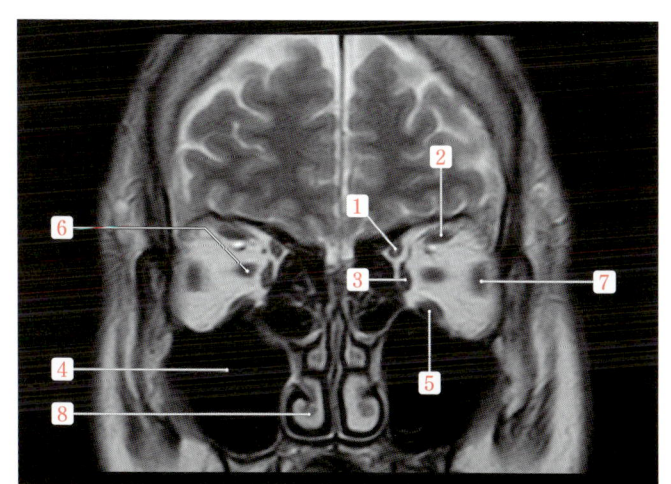

MRI T2強調像（冠状断像）

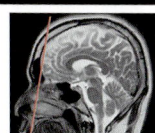

1 上斜筋　Superior oblique
2 上直筋　Superior rectus
3 内側直筋　Medial rectus
4 上顎洞　Maxillary sinus
5 下直筋　Inferior rectus
6 視神経　Optic nerve
7 外側直筋　Lateral rectus
8 下鼻甲介　Inferior nasal concha

頭頸部
Neck

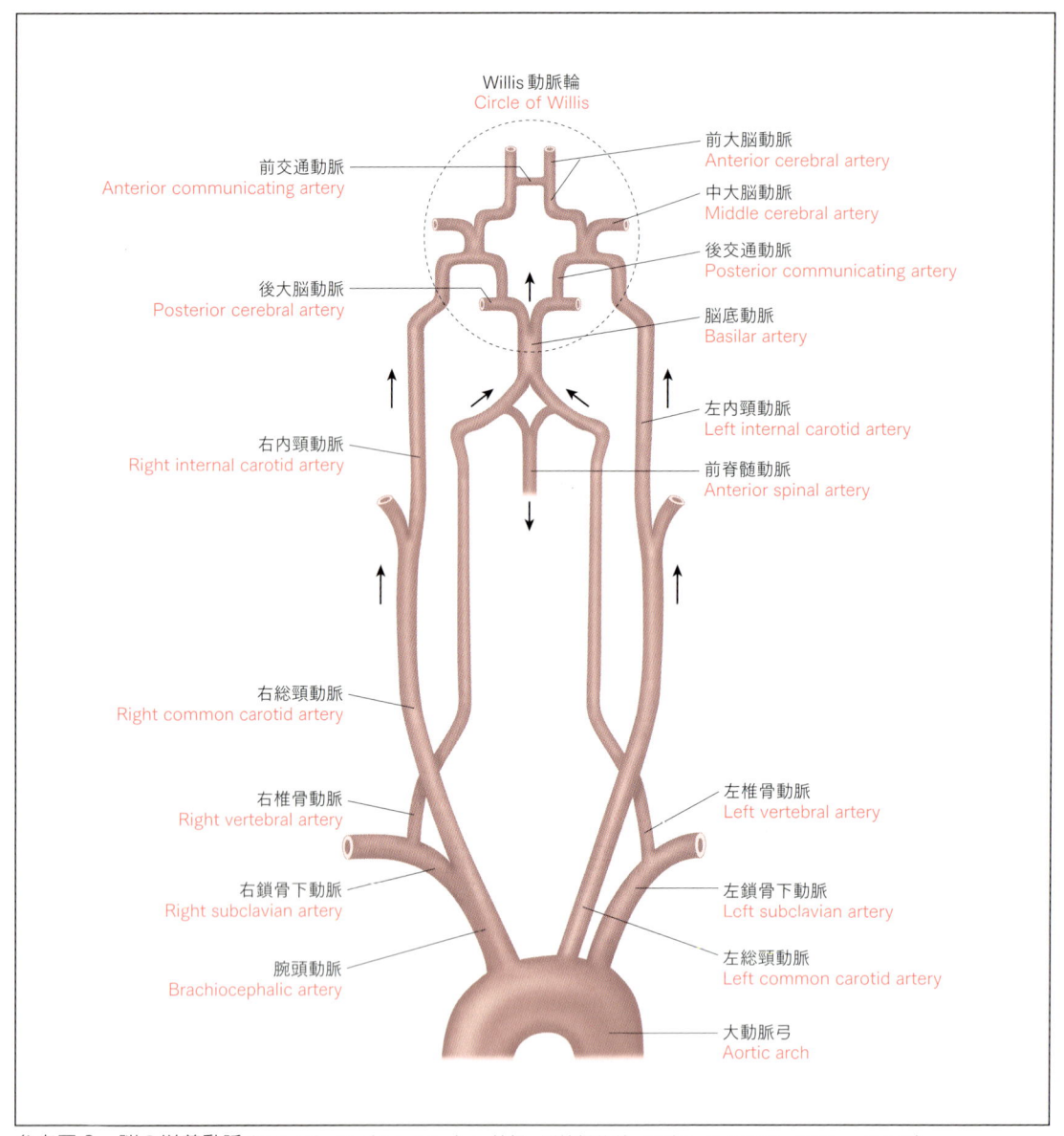

参考図3 脳の栄養動脈（アイメディスン〈iMedicine〉4．神経・脳神経外科．リブロ・サイエンス，2009，p.45より）

CT・MRI 解体新書

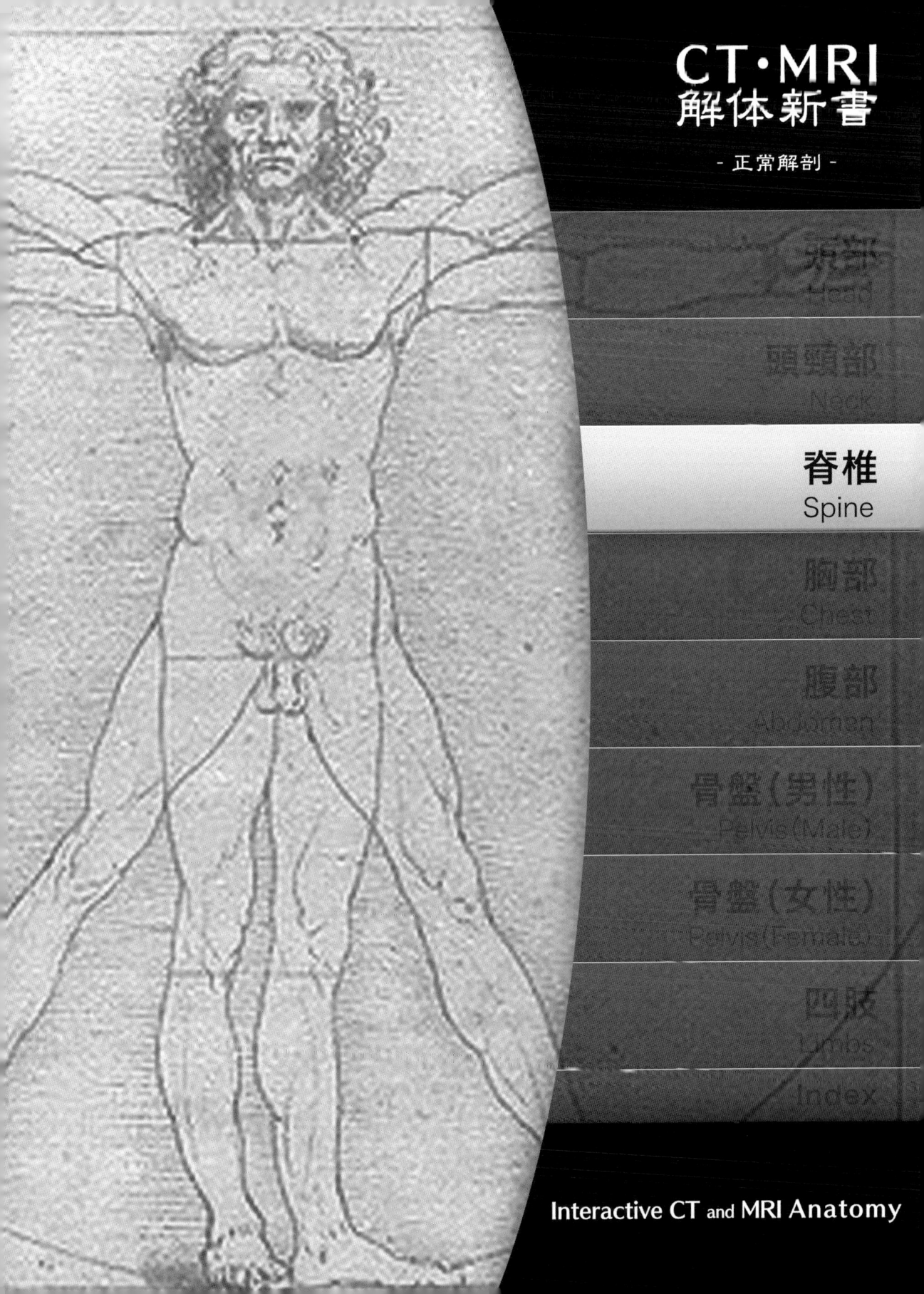

- 正常解剖 -

頭部
Head

頭頸部
Neck

脊椎
Spine

胸部
Chest

腹部
Abdomen

骨盤(男性)
Pelvis(Male)

骨盤(女性)
Pelvis(Female)

四肢
Limbs

Index

Interactive CT and MRI Anatomy

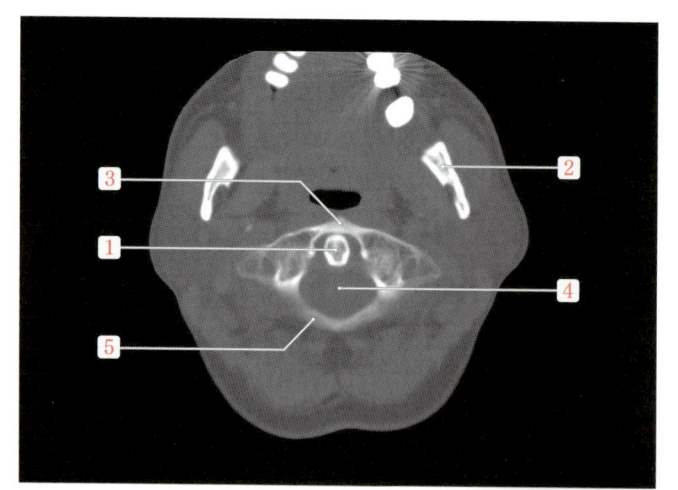

脊 椎
Spine

1 軸椎歯突起　Odontoid process
2 下顎骨　Mandible
3 環椎前弓　Anterior arch of atlas
4 脊柱管　Spinal canal
5 環椎後弓　Posterior arch of atlas

単純CT（横断像）

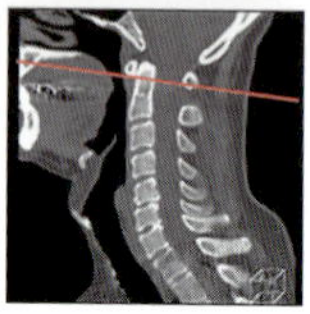

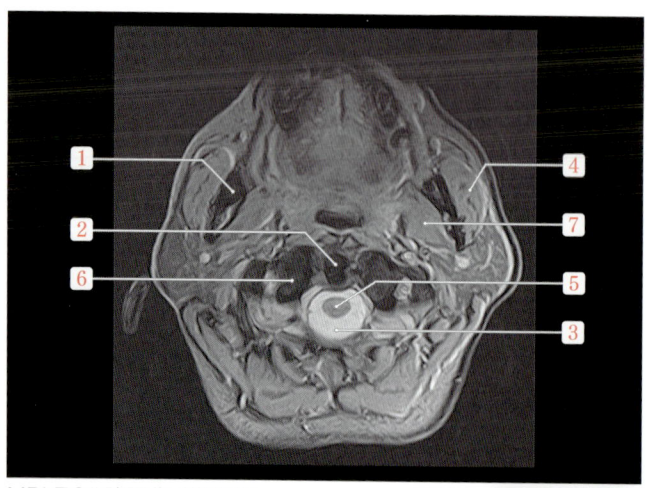

1 下顎骨　Mandible
2 軸椎歯突起　Odontoid process
3 脳脊髄液（クモ膜下腔）
　 Cerebrospinal fluid (Subarachnoid space)
4 咬筋　Masseter
5 脊髄　Spinal cord
6 環椎外側塊　Lateral mass of atlas
7 内側翼突筋　Medial pterygoid

MRI T2*強調像（横断像）

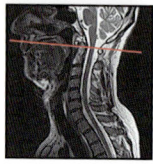

● CT・MRI解体新書

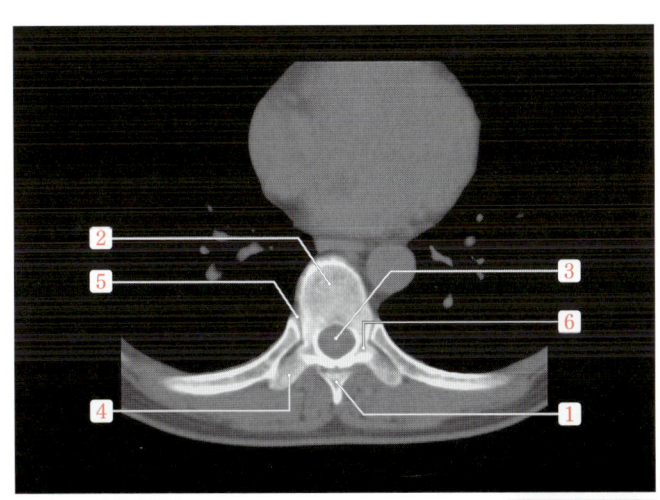

1 棘突起　Spinous process
2 椎体　Vertebral body
3 脊柱管　Spinal canal
4 横突起　Transverse process
5 肋椎関節　Costovertebral joint
6 椎弓根　Pedicle

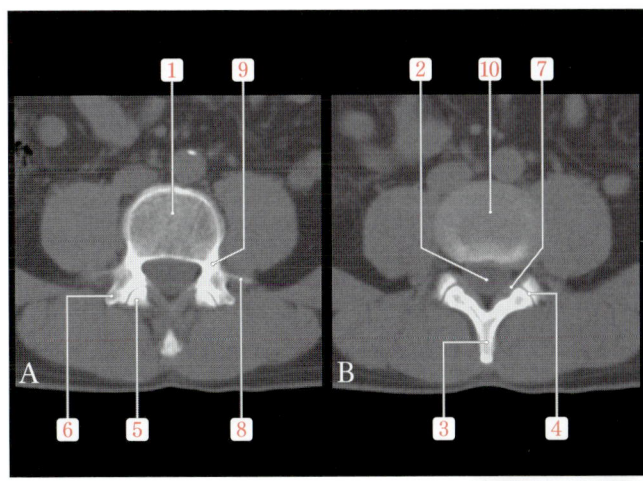

単純CT（横断像）

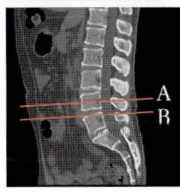

1 椎体　Vertebral body
2 脊柱管　Spinal canal
3 棘突起　Spinous process
4 椎間関節　Facet joint
5 下関節突起　Inferior articular process
6 上関節突起　Superior articular process
7 黄色靱帯　Yellow ligament
8 横突起　Transverse process
9 椎弓根　Pedicle
10 椎間板　Intervertebral disc

単純CT（横断像）

脊椎

35

脊椎
Spine

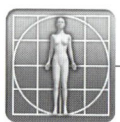

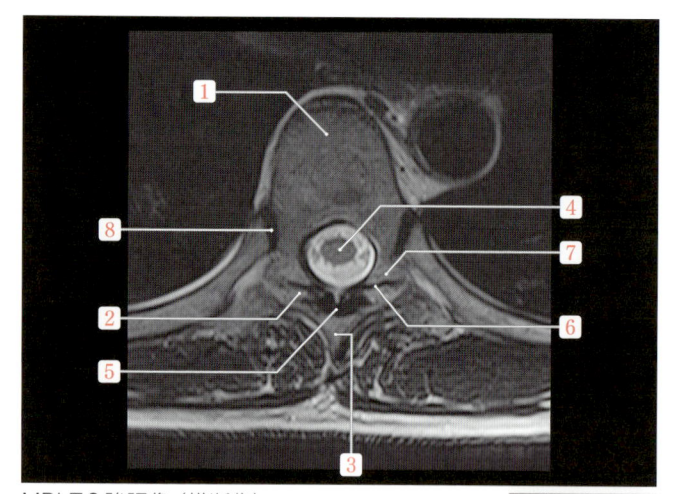

MRI T2強調像（横断像）

1 椎体　Vertebral body
2 椎弓　Vertebral arch
3 棘突起　Spinous process
4 脊髄　Spinal cord
5 黄色靱帯　Yellow ligament
6 椎間関節　Facet joint
7 椎弓根　Pedicle
8 肋椎関節　Costovertebral joint

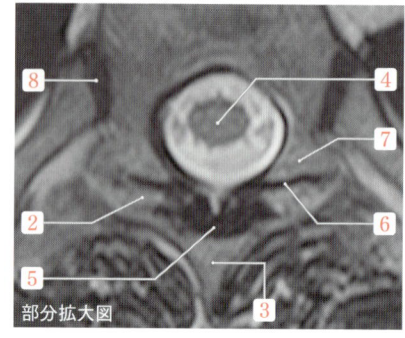

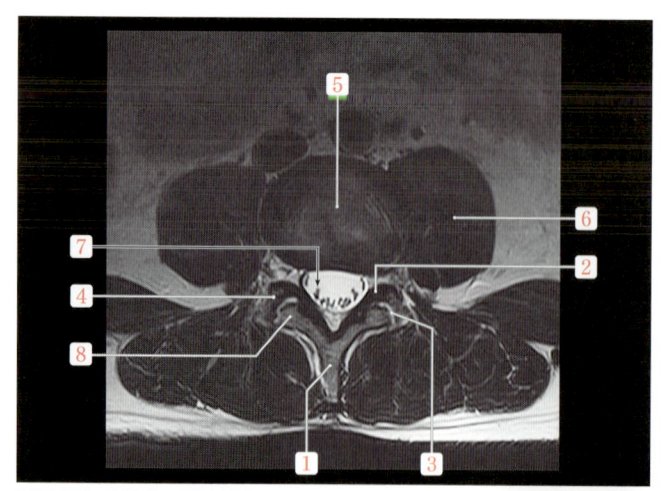

部分拡大図

MRI T2強調像（横断像）

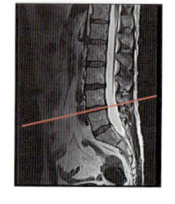

1 棘突起　Spinous process
2 黄色靱帯　Yellow ligament
3 椎間関節　Facet joint
4 上関節突起　Superior articular process
5 椎間板　Intervertebral disc
6 大腰筋　Psoas major
7 馬尾　Cauda equina
8 下関節突起　Inferior articular process

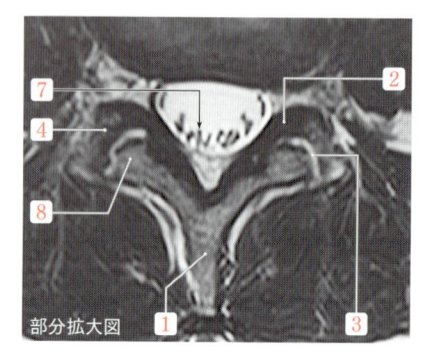

部分拡大図

36

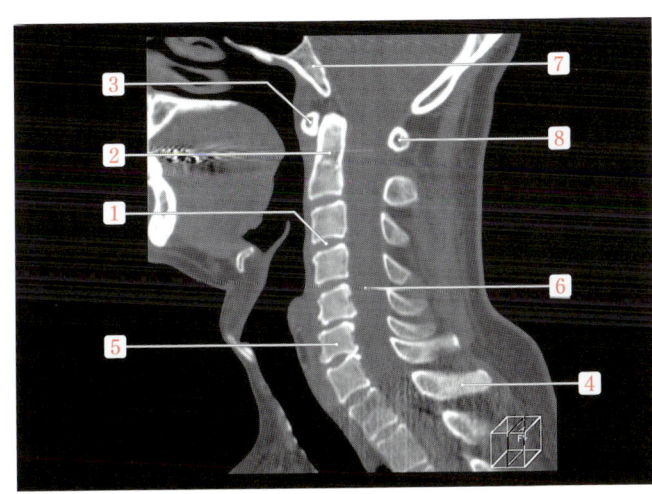

単純CT（正中矢状断像）

1 椎間板腔　Intervertebral disc space
2 軸椎歯突起　Odontoid process
3 環椎前弓　Anterior arch of atlas
4 棘突起　Spinous process
5 椎体　Vertebral body
6 脊柱管　Spinal canal
7 斜台　Clivus
8 環椎後弓　Posterior arch of atlas

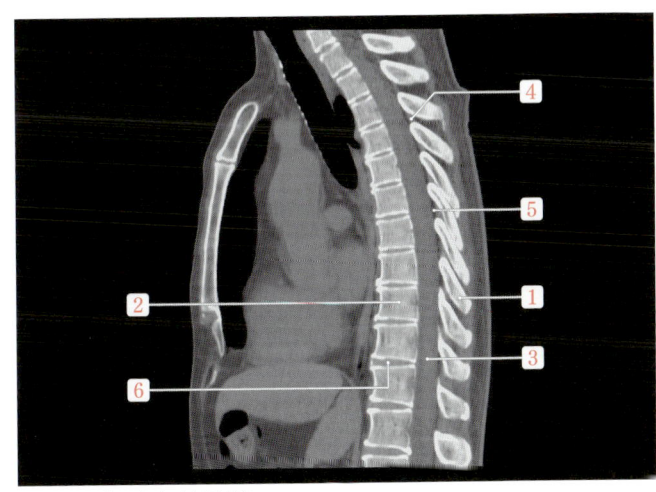

脊椎

単純CT（正中矢状断像）

1 棘突起　Spinous process
2 椎体　Vertebral body
3 脊柱管　Spinal canal
4 黄色靱帯　Yellow ligament
5 硬膜外脂肪　Epidural fat
6 椎間板腔　Intervertebral disc space

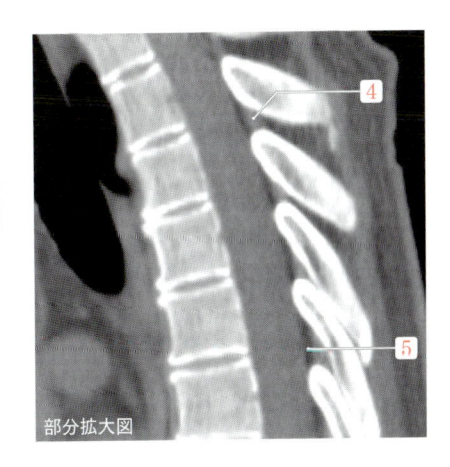

部分拡大図

脊椎
Spine

1 椎間板腔　Intervertebral disc space
2 椎体　Vertebral body
3 棘突起　Spinous process
4 硬膜外脂肪　Epidural fat
5 仙骨　Sacrum
6 脊柱管　Spinal canal

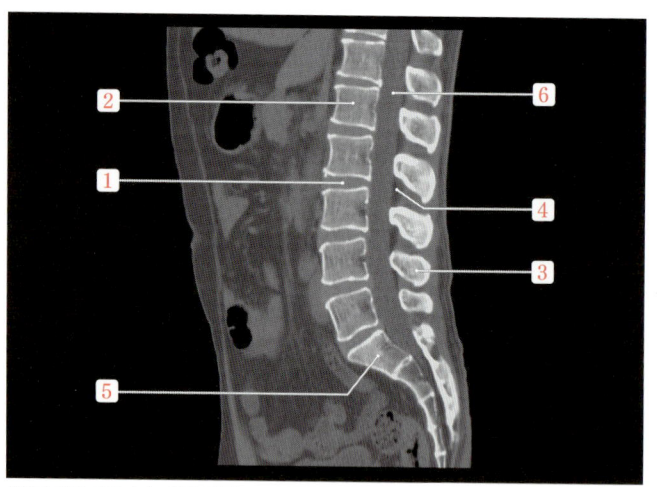

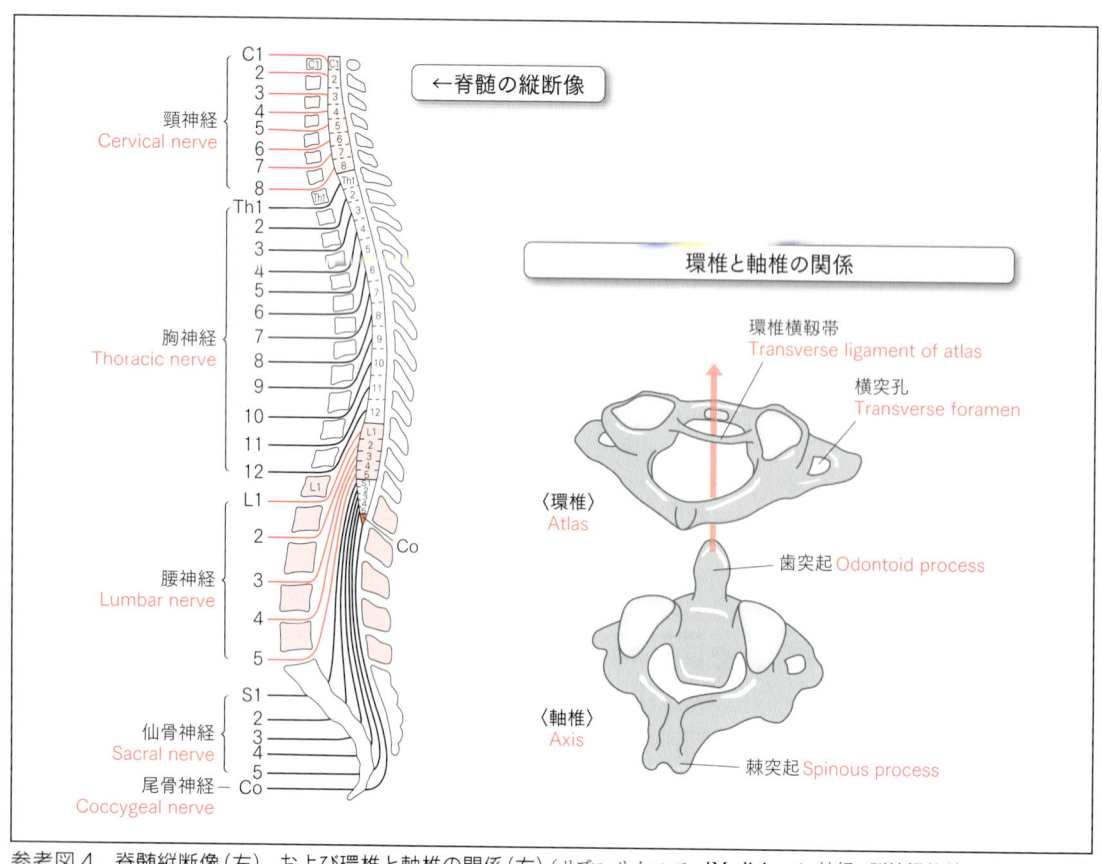

単純CT（正中矢状断像）

←脊髄の縦断像

頸神経 Cervical nerve
胸神経 Thoracic nerve
腰神経 Lumbar nerve
仙骨神経 Sacral nerve
尾骨神経 Coccygeal nerve

環椎と軸椎の関係

環椎横靱帯 Transverse ligament of atlas
横突孔 Transverse foramen
〈環椎〉Atlas
歯突起 Odontoid process
〈軸椎〉Axis
棘突起 Spinous process

参考図4　脊髄縦断像（左）、および環椎と軸椎の関係（右）（リブロ・サイエンス, iMedicine 4. 神経・脳神経外科, p.23・24 より）

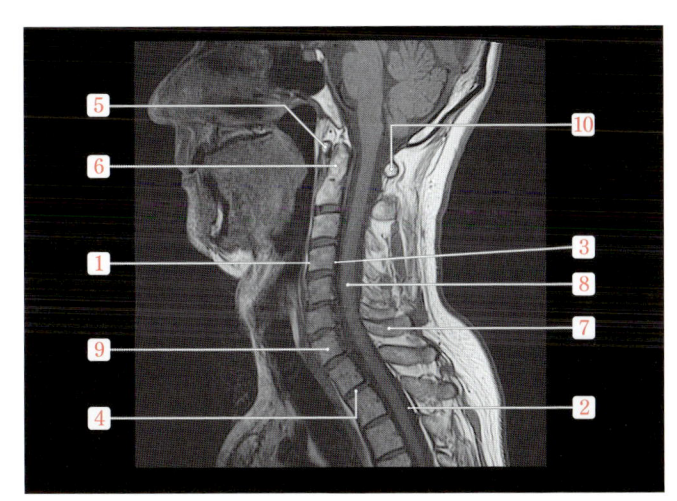

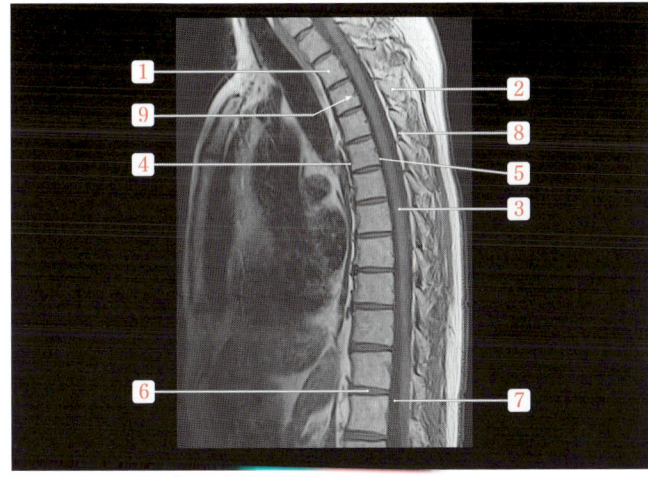

1 前縦靱帯　Anterior longitudinal ligament
2 脳脊髄液（クモ膜下腔）
　Cerebrospinal fluid (Subarachnoid space)
3 後縦靱帯　Posterior longitudinal ligament
4 椎間板　Intervertebral disc
5 環椎前弓　Anterior arch of atlas
6 軸椎歯突起　Odontoid process
7 棘突起　Spinous process
8 脊髄　Spinal cord
9 椎体　Vertebral body
10 環椎後弓　Posterior arch of atlas

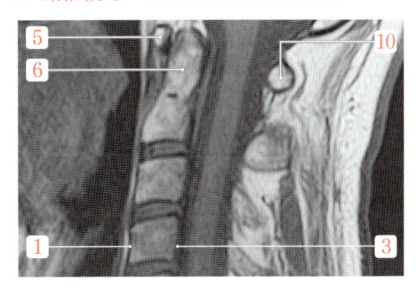

MRI T1強調像（正中矢状断像）

1 椎体　Vertebral body
2 棘突起　Spinous process
3 脊髄　Spinal cord
4 前縦靱帯　Anterior longitudinal ligament
5 後縦靱帯　Posterior longitudinal ligament
6 椎間板　Intervertebral disc
7 脳脊髄液　Cerebrospinal fluid
8 黄色靱帯　Yellow ligament
9 椎体静脈　Basivertebral vein

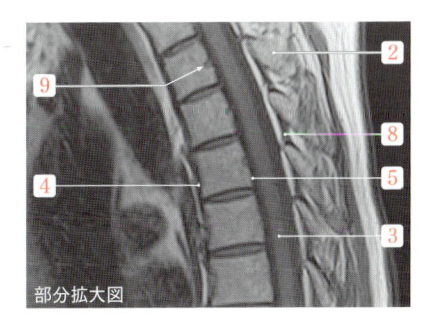

MRI T1強調像（正中矢状断像）

部分拡大図

脊椎

39

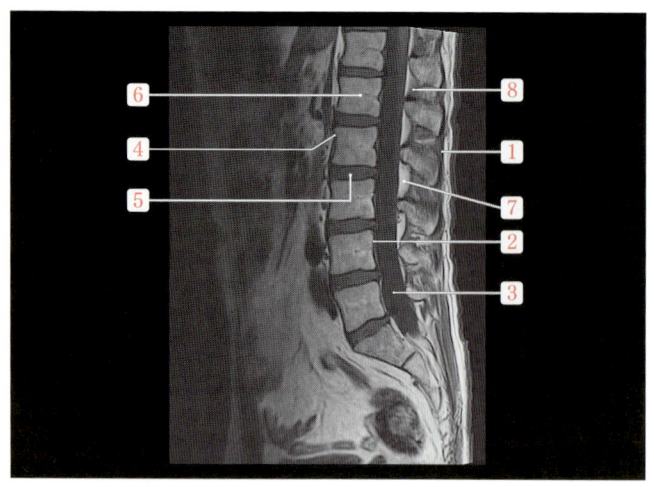

脊 椎
Spine

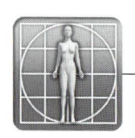

MRI T1強調像（正中矢状断像）

1 棘上靱帯　Supraspinous ligament
2 後縦靱帯　Posterior longitudinal ligament
3 脳脊髄液　Cerebrospinal fluid
4 前縦靱帯　Anterior longitudinal ligament
5 椎間板　Intervertebral disc
6 椎体　Vertebral body
7 硬膜外脂肪　Epidural fat
8 黄色靱帯　Yellow ligament

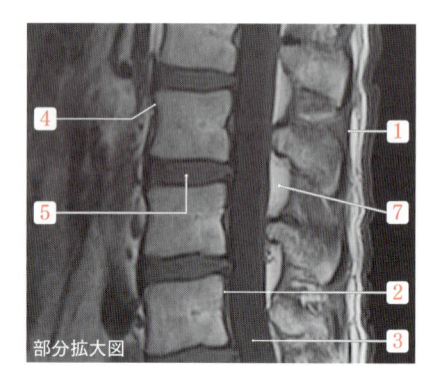

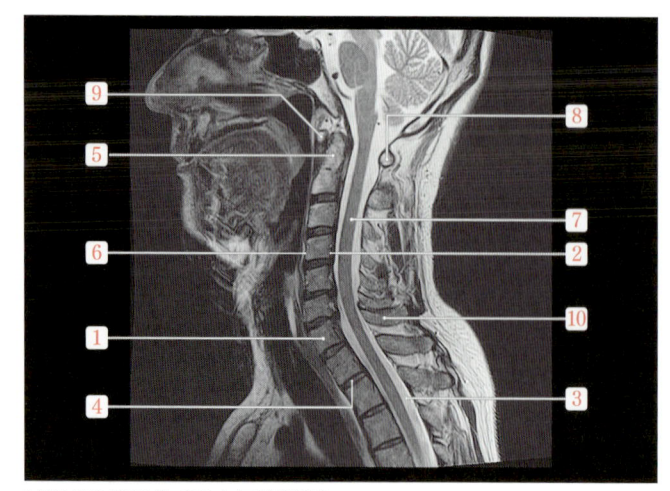

部分拡大図

MRI T2強調像（正中矢状断像）

1 椎体　Vertebral body
2 後縦靱帯　Posterior longitudinal ligament
3 脳脊髄液（クモ膜下腔）
　Cerebrospinal fluid (Subarachnoid space)
4 椎間板　Intervertebral disc
5 軸椎歯突起　Odontoid process
6 前縦靱帯　Anterior longitudinal ligament
7 脊髄　Spinal cord
8 環椎後弓　Posterior arch of atlas
9 環椎前弓　Anterior arch of atlas
10 棘突起　Spinous process

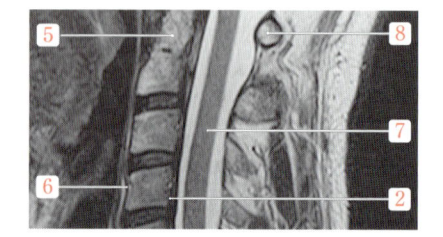

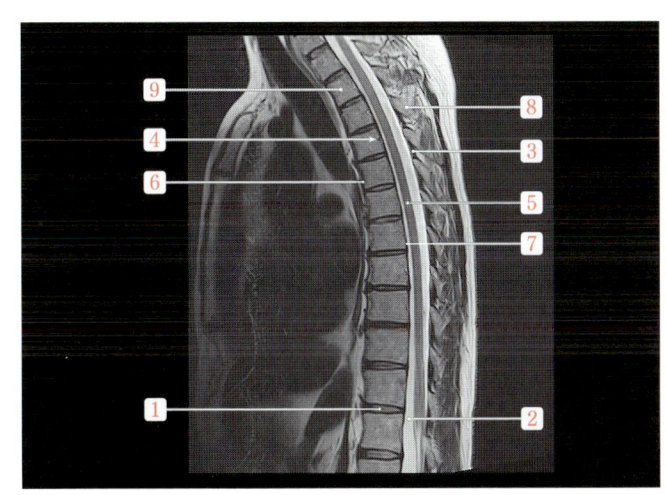

● CT・MRI 解体新書

1 椎間板　Intervertebral disc
2 脳脊髄液　Cerebrospinal fluid
3 黄色靱帯　Yellow ligament
4 椎体静脈　Basivertebral vein
5 脊髄　Spinal cord
6 前縦靱帯　Anterior longitudinal ligament
7 後縦靱帯　Posterior longitudinal ligament
8 棘突起　Spinous process
9 椎体　Vertebral body

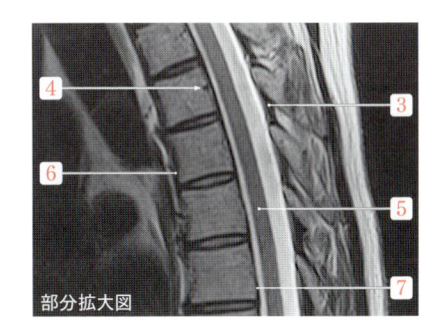

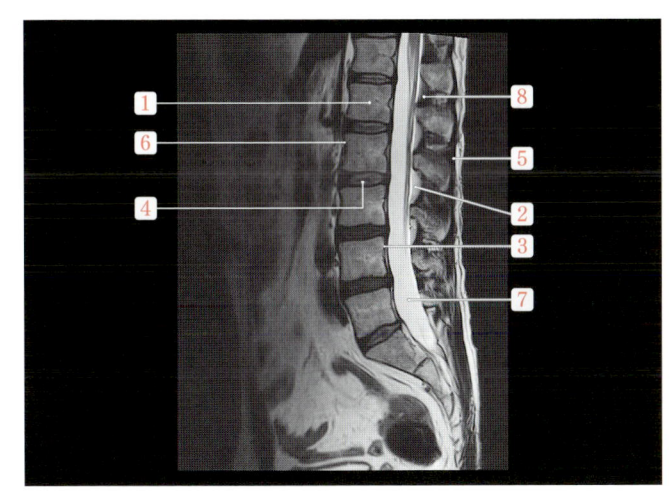

MRI T2強調像（正中矢状断像）

部分拡大図

1 椎体　Vertebral body
2 硬膜外脂肪　Epidural fat
3 後縦靱帯　Posterior longitudinal ligament
4 椎間板　Intervertebral disc
5 棘上靱帯　Supraspinous ligament
6 前縦靱帯　Anterior longitudinal ligament
7 脳脊髄液　Cerebrospinal fluid
8 黄色靱帯　Yellow ligament

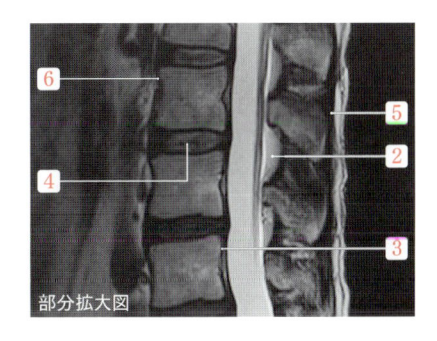

MRI T2強調像（正中矢状断像）

部分拡大図

脊椎

41

脊 椎
Spine

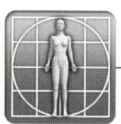

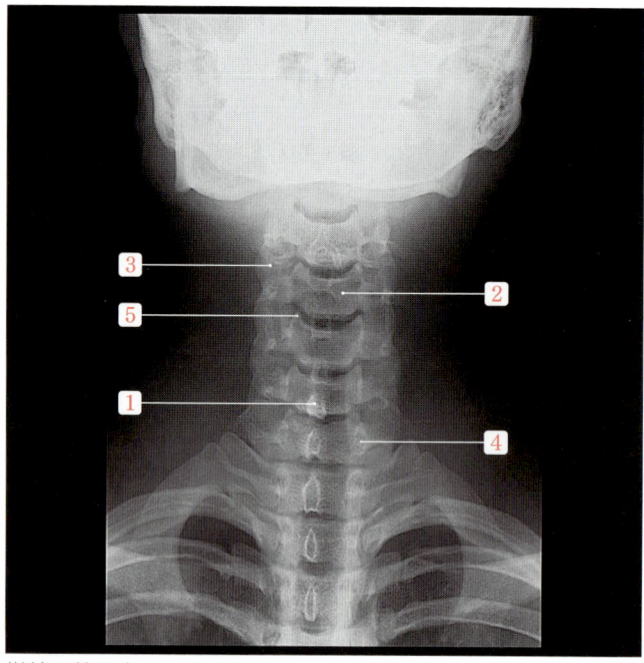

単純X線写真正面像（頸椎）

1 棘突起　Spinous process
2 椎体　Vertebral body
3 椎間関節　Intervertebral joint
4 椎弓根　Pedicle
5 鉤状突起　Uncinate process

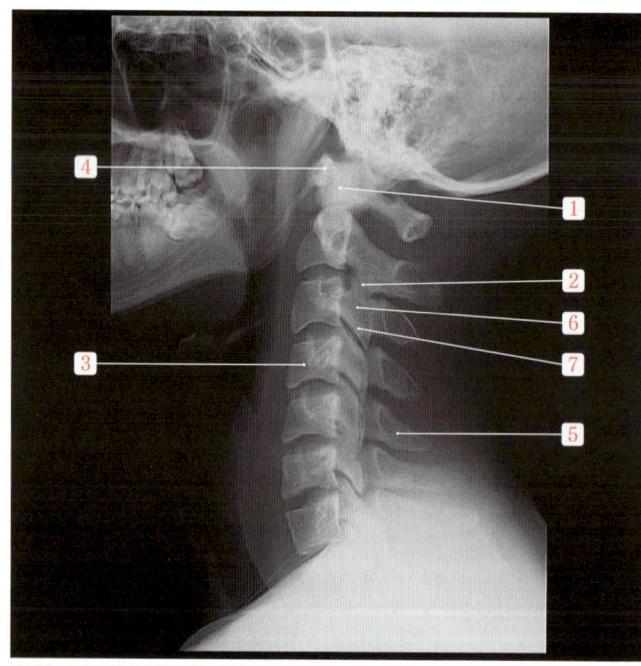

単純X線写真側面像（頸椎）

1 軸椎歯突起　Odontoid process
2 上関節突起　Superior articular process
3 椎体　Vertebral body
4 環椎前弓　Anterior arch of atlas
5 棘突起　Spinous process
6 椎間関節柱　Articular pillar
7 下関節突起　Inferior articular process

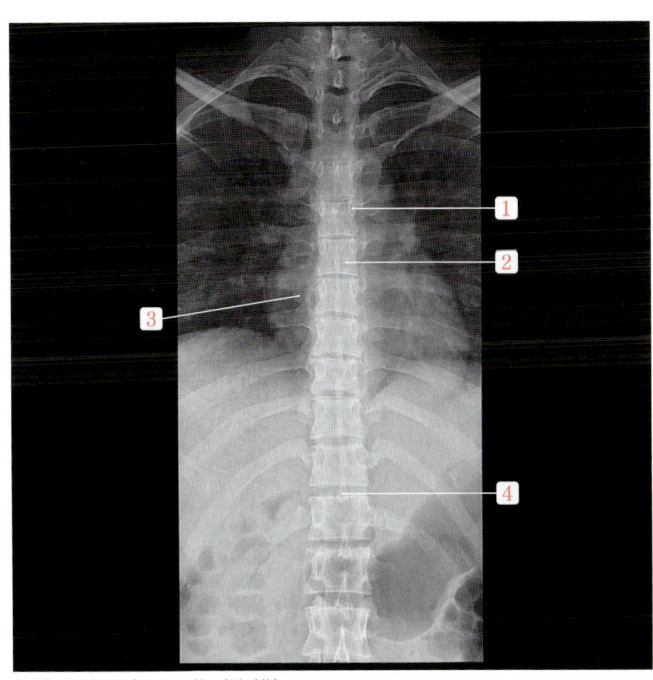

1 椎弓根　Pedicle
2 椎体　Vertebral body
3 横突起　Transverse process
4 棘突起　Spinous process

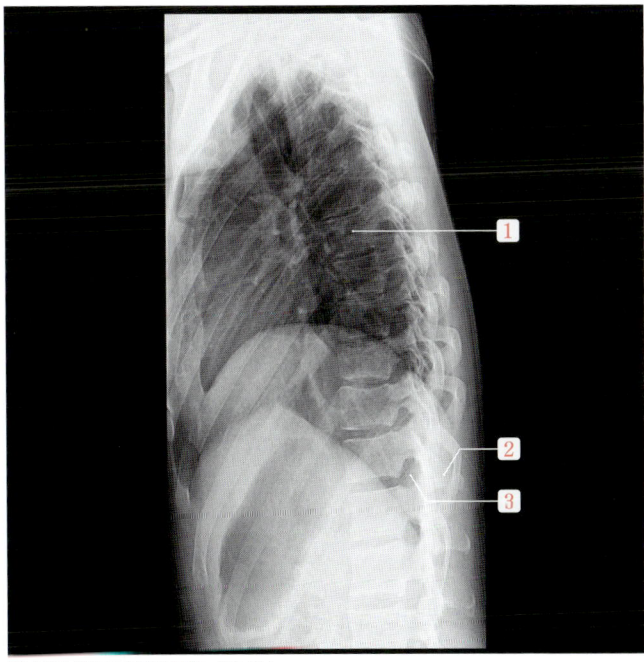

単純X線写真正面像（胸椎）

1 椎体　Vertebral body
2 棘突起　Spinous process
3 椎間孔　Intervertebral foramen

単純X線写真側面像（胸椎）

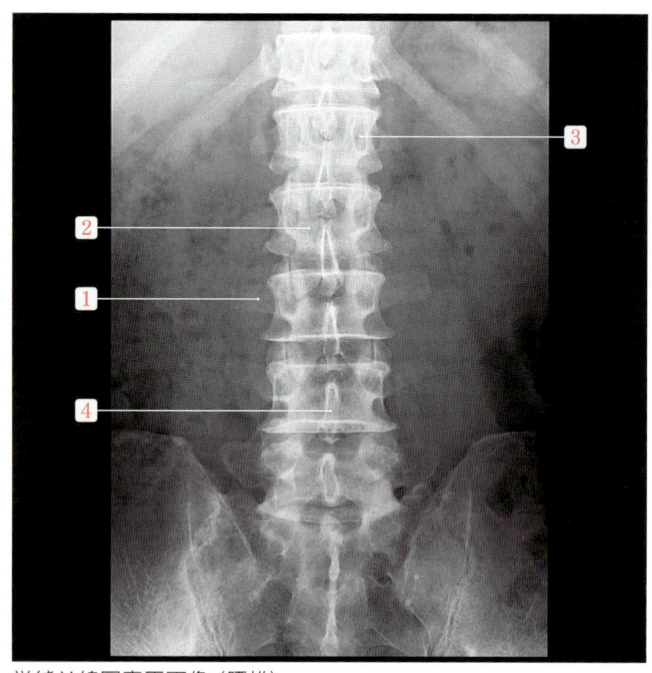

脊 椎
Spine

1 横突起　Transverse process
2 椎体　Vertebral body
3 椎弓根　Pedicle
4 棘突起　Spinous process

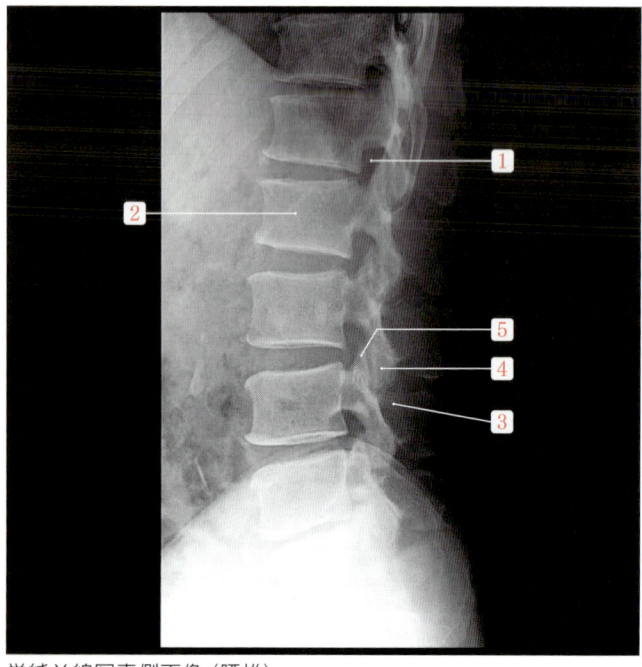

単純X線写真正面像（腰椎）

1 椎間孔　Intervertebral foramen
2 椎体　Vertebral body
3 棘突起　Spinous process
4 下関節突起　Inferior articular process
5 上関節突起　Superior articular process

単純X線写真側面像（腰椎）

CT・MRI
解体新書

- 正常解剖 -

頭部 / Head

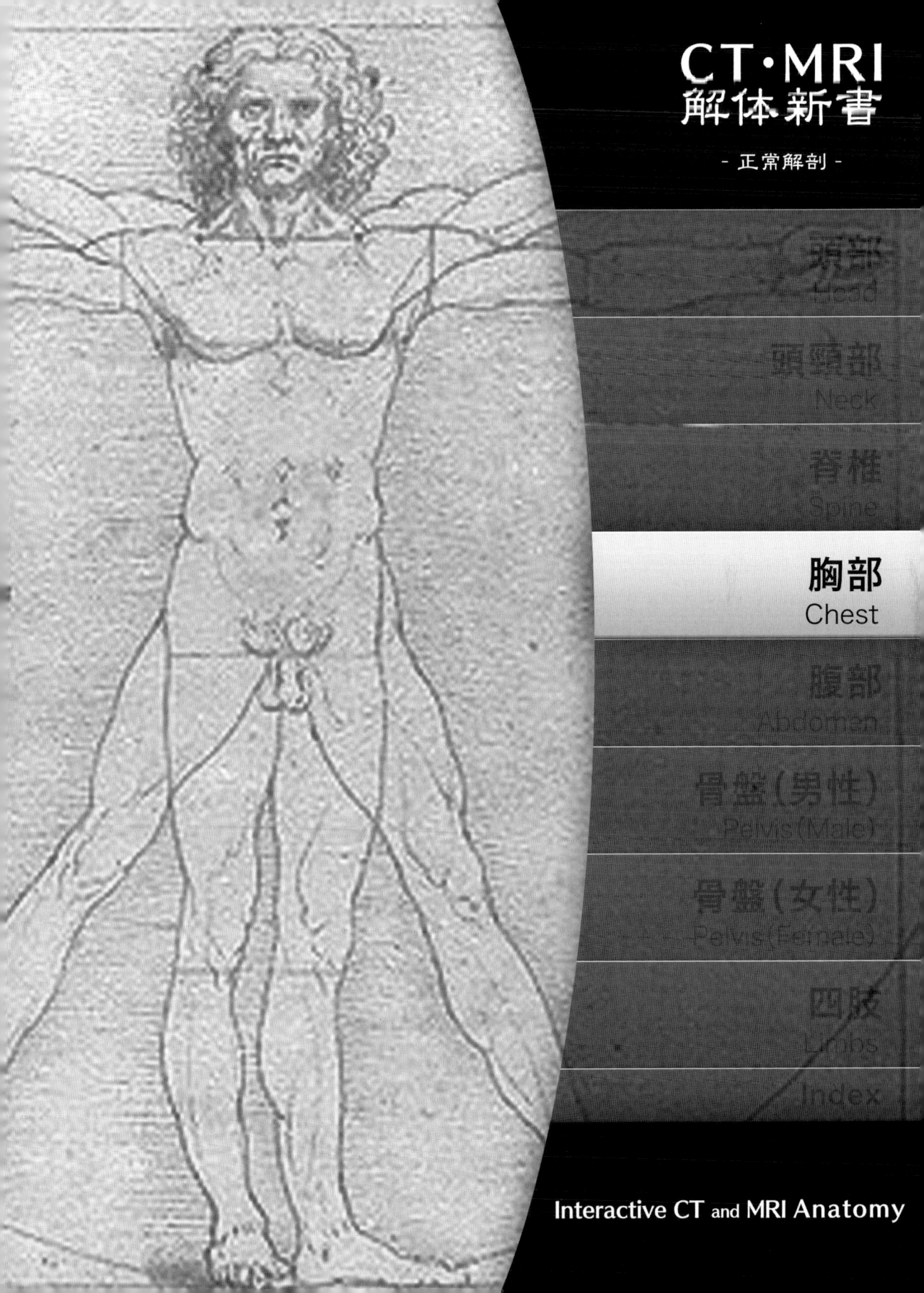

頭頸部 / Neck

脊椎 / Spine

胸部
Chest

腹部 / Abdomen

骨盤(男性) / Pelvis (Male)

骨盤(女性) / Pelvis (Female)

四肢 / Limbs

Index

Interactive CT and MRI Anatomy

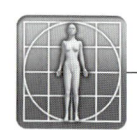

胸 部
Chest

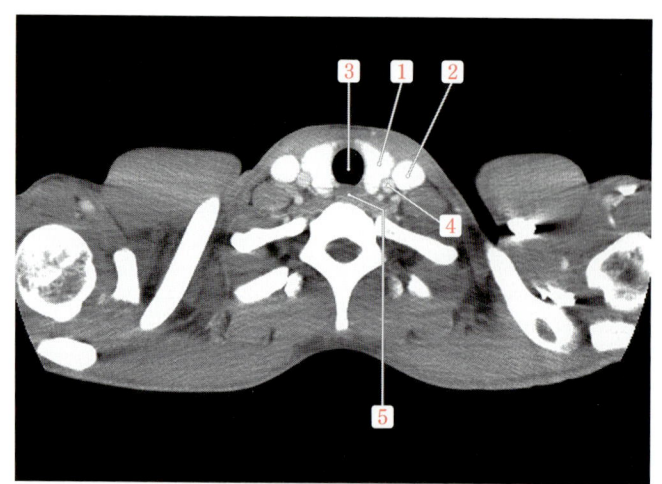

造影CT（縦隔条件、横断像）

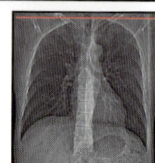

1 甲状腺　Thyroid gland
2 内頸静脈　Internal jugular vein
3 気管　Trachea
4 総頸動脈　Common carotid artery
5 食道　Esophagus

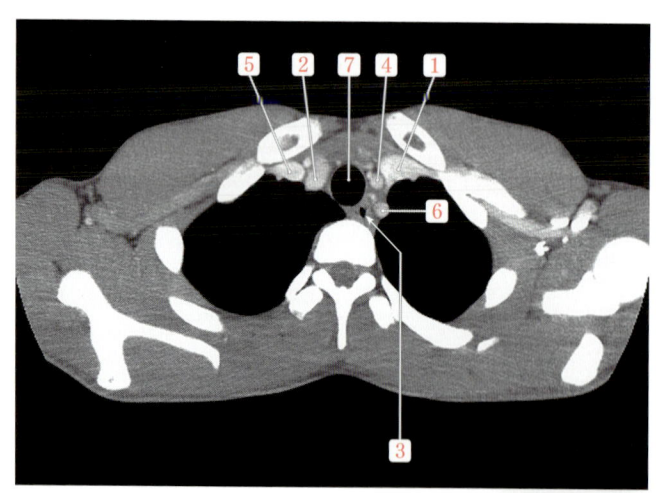

造影CT（縦隔条件、横断像）

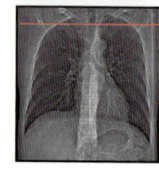

1 左腕頭静脈　Left brachiocephalic vein
2 腕頭動脈　Brachiocephalic artery
3 食道　Esophagus
4 左総頸動脈　Left common carotid artery
5 右腕頭静脈　Right brachiocephalic vein
6 左鎖骨下動脈　Left subclavian artery
7 気管　Trachea

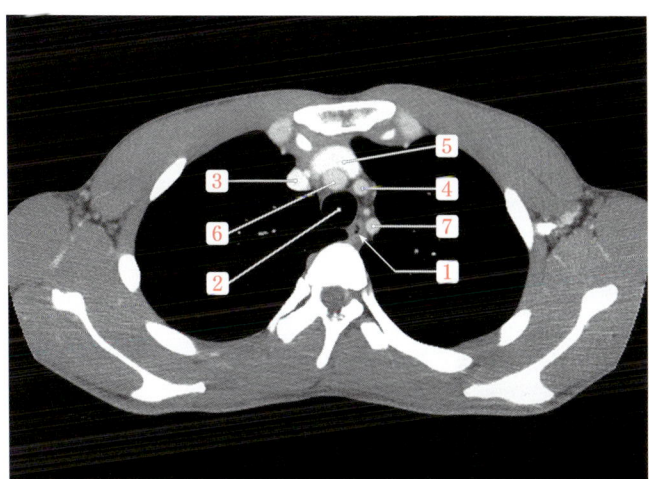

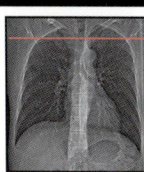

1 食道　Esophagus
2 気管　Trachea
3 右腕頭静脈　Right brachiocephalic vein
4 左総頸動脈　Left common carotid artery
5 左腕頭静脈　Left brachiocephalic vein
6 腕頭動脈　Brachiocephalic artery
7 左鎖骨下動脈　Left subclavian artery

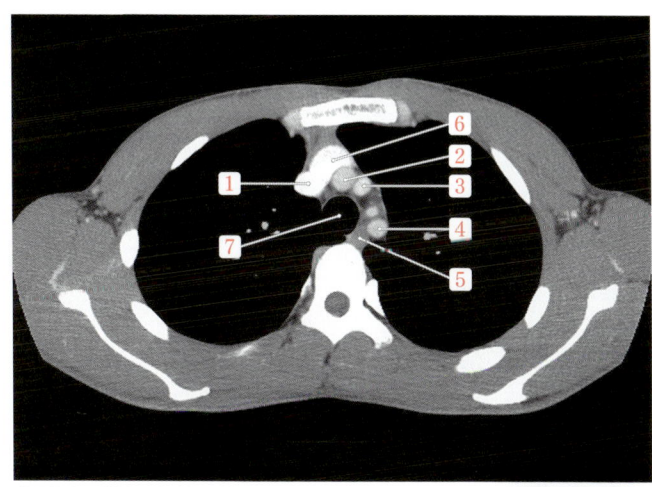

造影CT（縦隔条件、横断像）

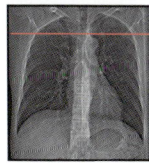

1 右腕頭静脈　Right brachiocephalic vein
2 腕頭動脈　Brachiocephalic artery
3 左総頸動脈　Left common carotid artery
4 左鎖骨下動脈　Left subclavian artery
5 食道　Esophagus
6 左腕頭静脈　Left brachiocephalic vein
7 気管　Trachea

造影CT（縦隔条件、横断像）

胸部

47

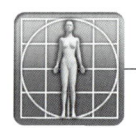

胸 部
Chest

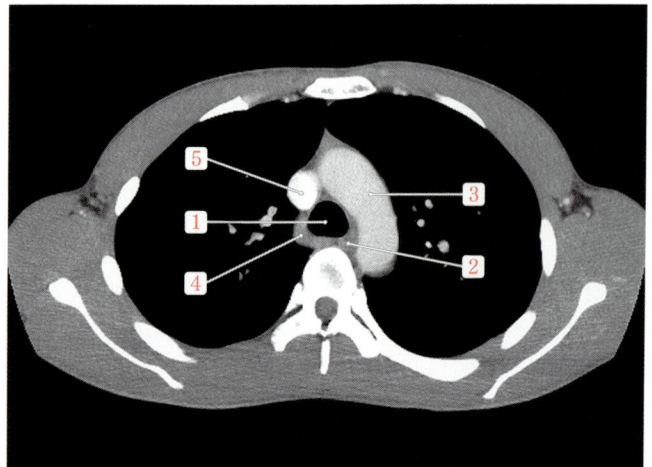

造影CT（縦隔条件、横断像）

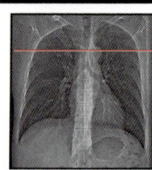

1　気管　Trachea
2　食道　Esophagus
3　大動脈弓　Aortic arch
4　奇静脈弓　Azygos arch
5　上大静脈　Superior vena cava

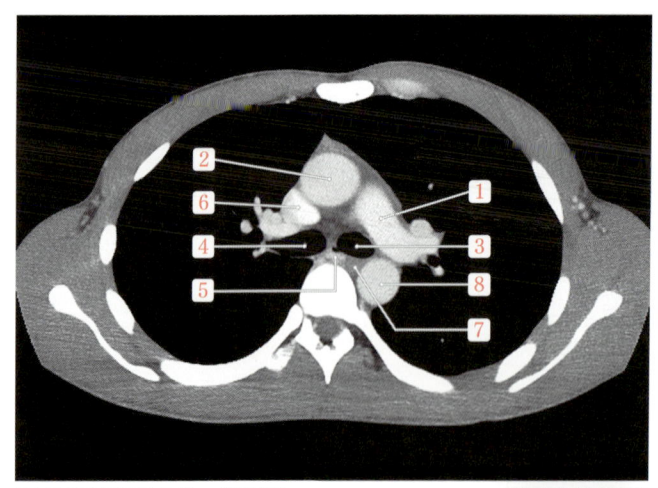

造影CT（縦隔条件、横断像）

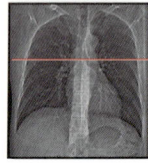

1　左肺動脈　Left pulmonary artery
2　上行大動脈　Ascending aorta
3　左主気管支　Left main bronchus
4　右主気管支　Right main bronchus
5　奇静脈　Azygos vein
6　上大静脈　Superior vena cava
7　食道　Esophagus
8　下行大動脈　Descending aorta

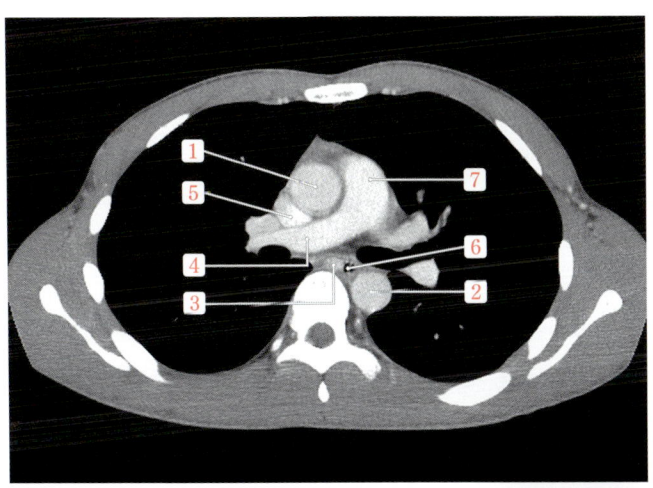

造影CT（縦隔条件、横断像）

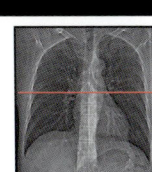

1 上行大動脈　Ascending aorta
2 下行大動脈　Descending aorta
3 奇静脈　Azygos vein
4 右肺動脈　Right pulmonary artery
5 上大静脈　Superior vena cava
6 食道　Esophagus
7 肺動脈幹　Pulmonary trunk

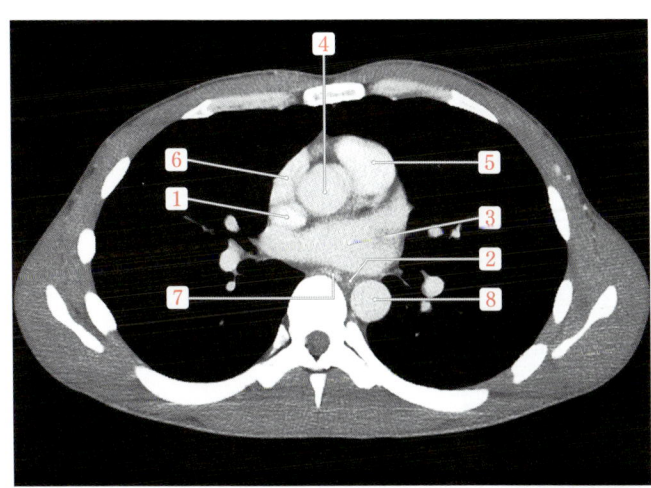

造影CT（縦隔条件、横断像）

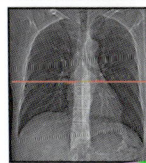

1 上大静脈　Superior vena cava
2 食道　Esophagus
3 左心房　Left atrium
4 大動脈弁　Aortic valve
5 肺動脈弁　Pulmonary valve
6 右心耳　Right auricle
7 奇静脈　Azygos vein
8 下行大動脈　Descending aorta

胸部

49

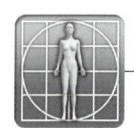

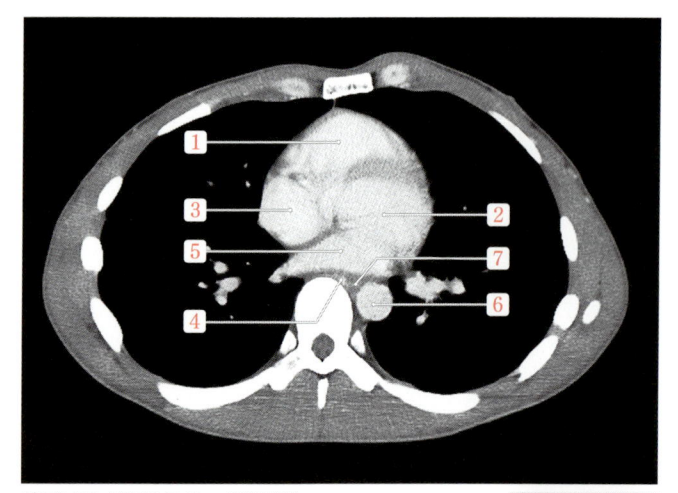

胸部
Chest

造影 CT（縦隔条件、横断像）

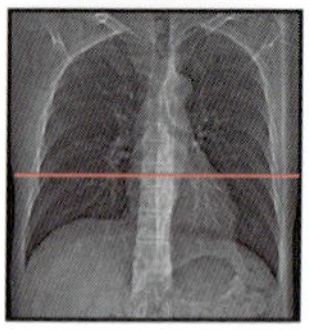

1 右心室　Right ventricle
2 左心室　Left ventricle
3 右心房　Right atrium
4 奇静脈　Azygos vein
5 左心房　Left atrium
6 下行大動脈　Descending aorta
7 食道　Esophagus

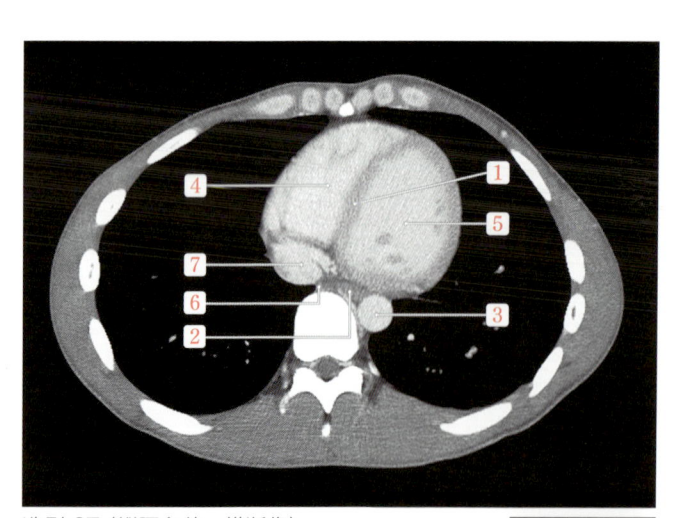

造影 CT（縦隔条件、横断像）

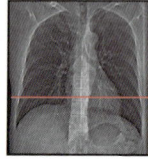

1 心室中隔　Interventricular septum
2 食道　Esophagus
3 下行大動脈　Descending aorta
4 右心室　Right ventricle
5 左心室　Left ventricle
6 奇静脈　Azygos vein
7 下大静脈　Inferior vena cava

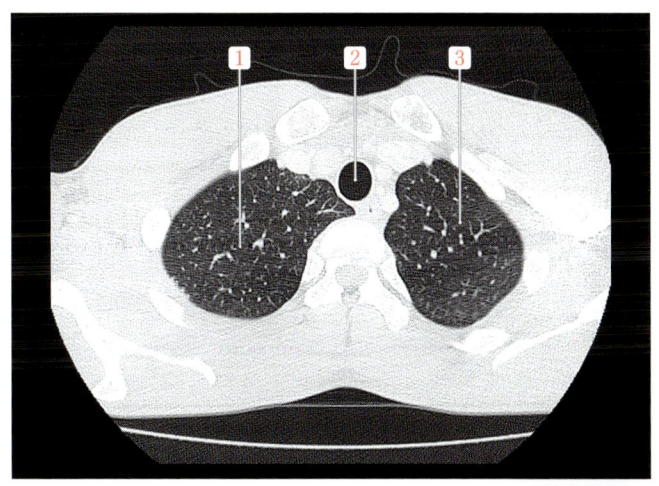

1 右肺上葉　Upper lobe of right lung
2 気管　Trachea
3 左肺上葉　Upper lobe of left lung

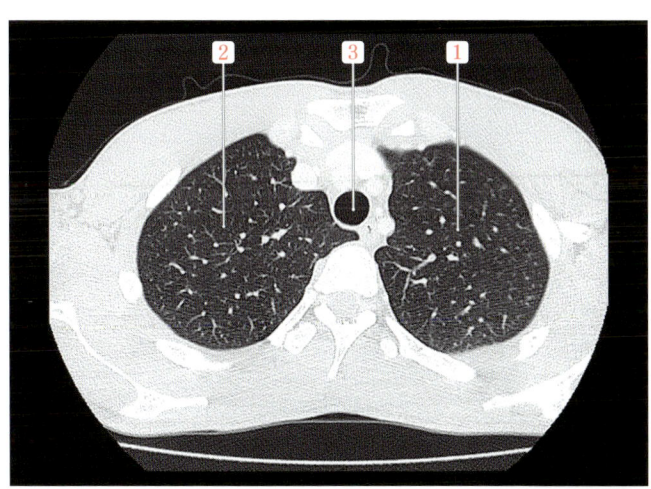

高分解能CT（肺野条件、横断像）

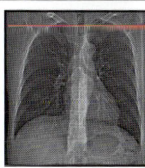

1 左肺上葉　Upper lobe of left lung
2 右肺上葉　Upper lobe of right lung
3 気管　Trachea

高分解能CT（肺野条件、横断像）

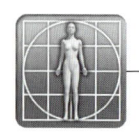

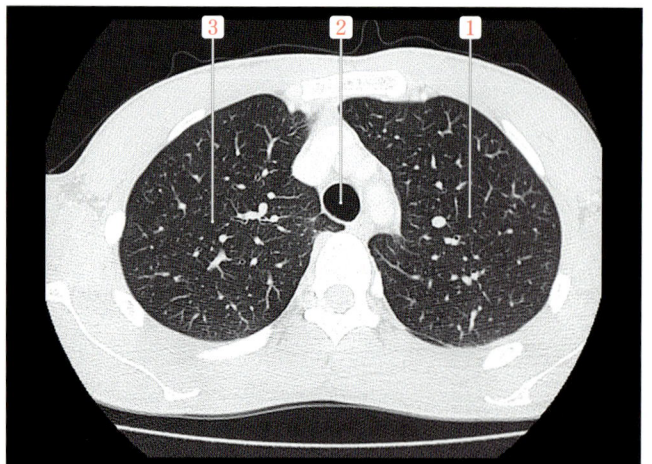

胸 部
Chest

1 左肺上葉　Upper lobe of left lung
2 気管　Trachea
3 右肺上葉　Upper lobe of right lung

高分解能CT（肺野条件、横断像）

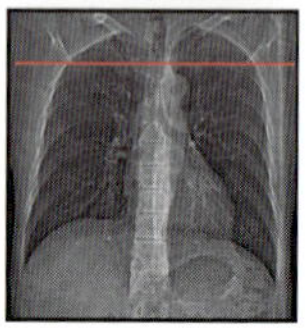

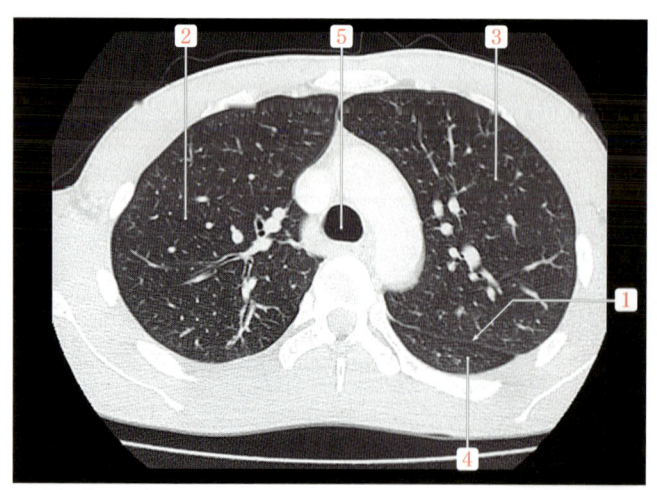

1 左大葉間裂　Left major fissure
2 右肺上葉　Upper lobe of right lung
3 左肺上葉　Upper lobe of left lung
4 左肺下葉　Lower lobe of left lung
5 気管　Trachea

高分解能CT（肺野条件、横断像）

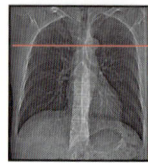

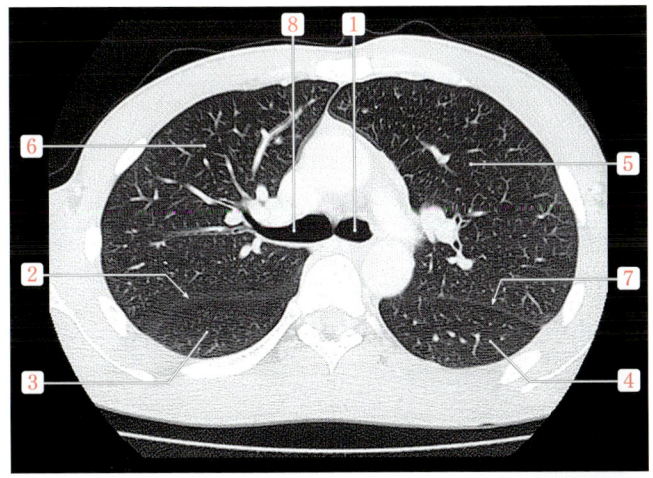

高分解能CT（肺野条件、横断像）

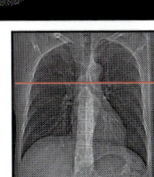

1 左主気管支　Left main bronchus
2 右大葉間裂　Right major fissure
3 右肺下葉　Lower lobe of right lung
4 左肺下葉　Lower lobe of left lung
5 左肺上葉　Upper lobe of left lung
6 右肺上葉　Upper lobe of right lung
7 左大葉間裂　Left major fissure
8 右主気管支　Right main bronchus

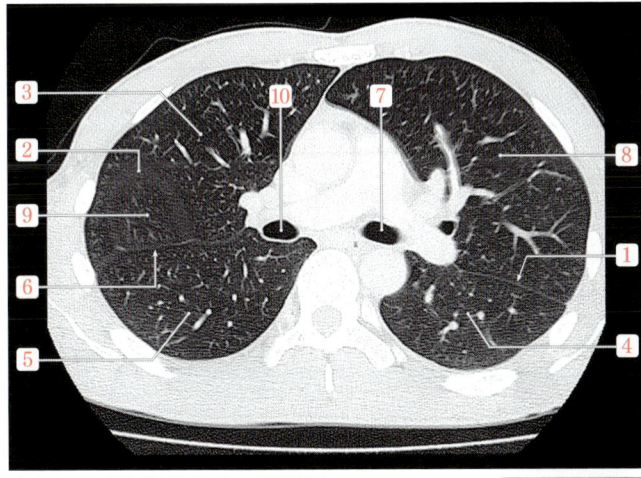

高分解能CT（肺野条件、横断像）

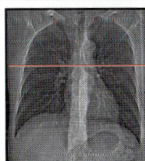

1 左大葉間裂　Left major fissure
2 小葉間裂　Minor fissure
3 右肺上葉　Upper lobe of right lung
4 左肺下葉　Lower lobe of left lung
5 右肺下葉　Lower lobe of right lung
6 右大葉間裂　Right major fissure
7 左主気管支　Left main bronchus
8 左肺上葉　Upper lobe of left lung
9 右肺中葉　Middle lobe of right lung
10 中間気管支幹　Truncus intermedius

胸部

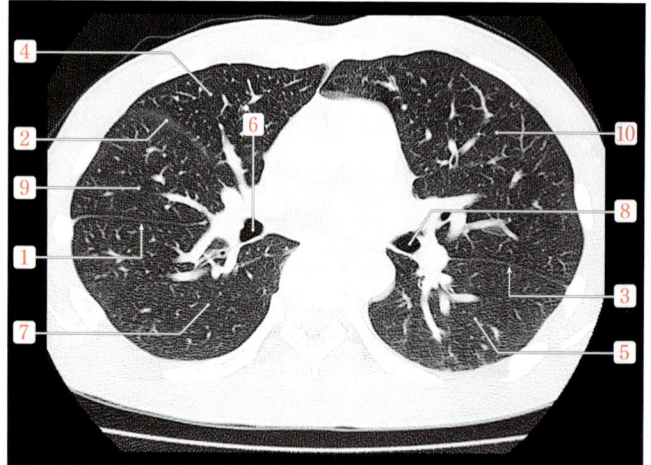

胸 部
Chest

高分解能CT（肺野条件、横断像）

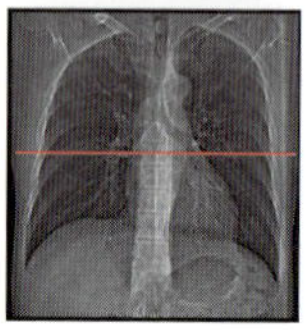

1 右大葉間裂　Right major fissure
2 小葉間裂　Minor fissure
3 左大葉間裂　Left major fissure
4 右肺上葉　Upper lobe of right lung
5 左肺下葉　Lower lobe of left lung
6 中間気管支幹　Truncus intermedius
7 右肺下葉　Lower lobe of right lung
8 左下葉気管支
　 Left inferior lobar bronchus
9 右肺中葉　Middle lobe of right lung
10 左肺上葉　Upper lobe of left lung

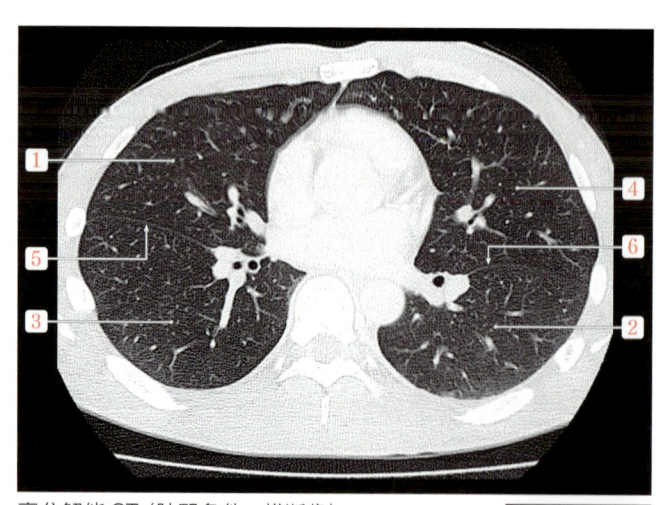

高分解能CT（肺野条件、横断像）

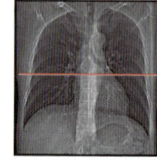

1 右肺中葉　Middle lobe of right lung
2 左肺下葉　Lower lobe of left lung
3 右肺下葉　Lower lobe of right lung
4 左肺上葉　Upper lobe of left lung
5 右大葉間裂　Right major fissure
6 左大葉間裂　Left major fissure

● CT・MRI 解体新書

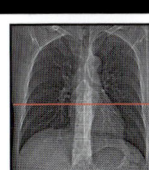

1 左肺上葉舌区　Lingular segment
2 右大葉間裂　Right major fissure
3 右肺中葉　Middle lobe of right lung
4 左肺下葉　Lower lobe of left lung
5 左大葉間裂　Left major fissure
6 右肺下葉　Lower lobe of right lung

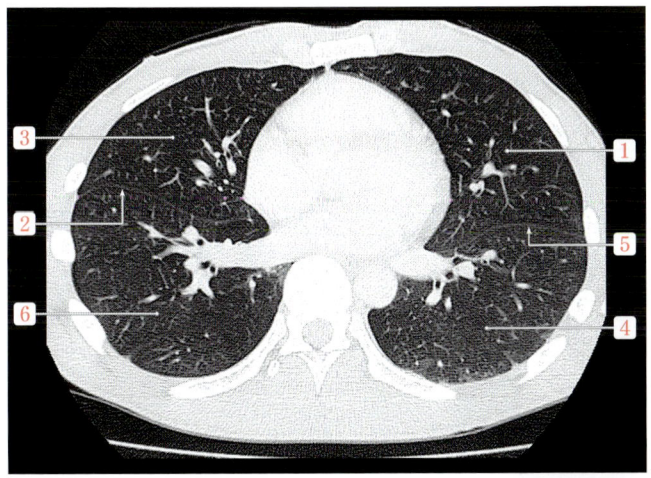

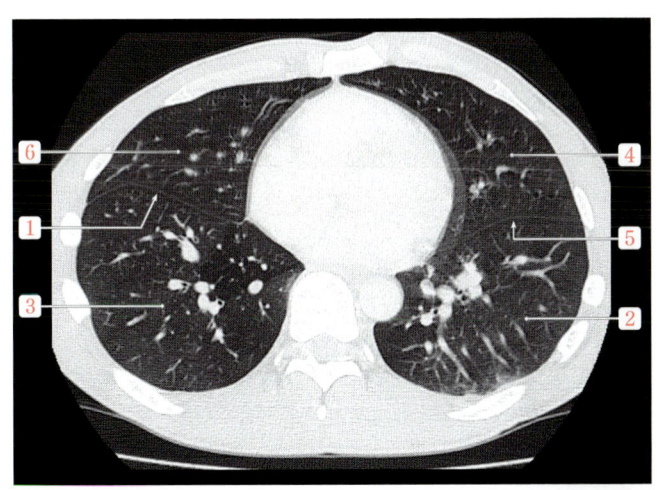

高分解能CT（肺野条件、横断像）

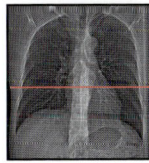

1 右大葉間裂　Right major fissure
2 左肺下葉　Lower lobe of left lung
3 右肺下葉　Lower lobe of right lung
4 左肺上葉舌区　Lingular segment
5 左大葉間裂　Left major fissure
6 右肺中葉　Middle lobe of right lung

高分解能CT（肺野条件、横断像）

胸部

55

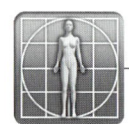

胸 部
Chest

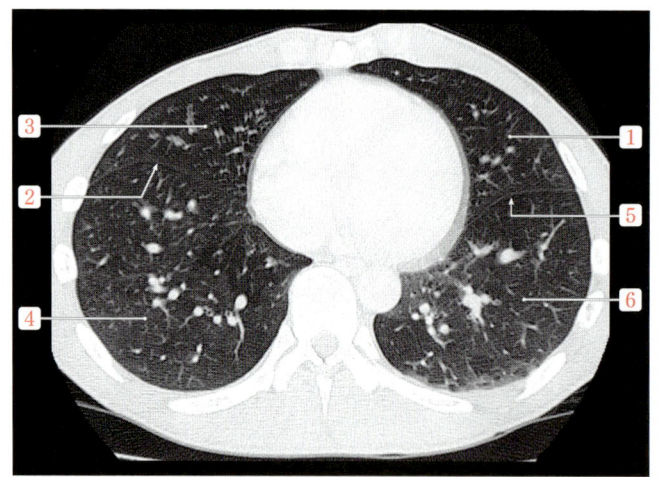

高分解能CT（肺野条件、横断像）

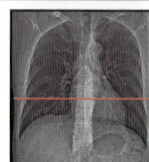

1 左肺上葉舌区　Lingular segment
2 右大葉間裂　Right major fissure
3 右肺中葉　Middle lobe of right lung
4 右肺下葉　Lower lobe of right lung
5 左大葉間裂　Left major fissure
6 左肺下葉　Lower lobe of left lung

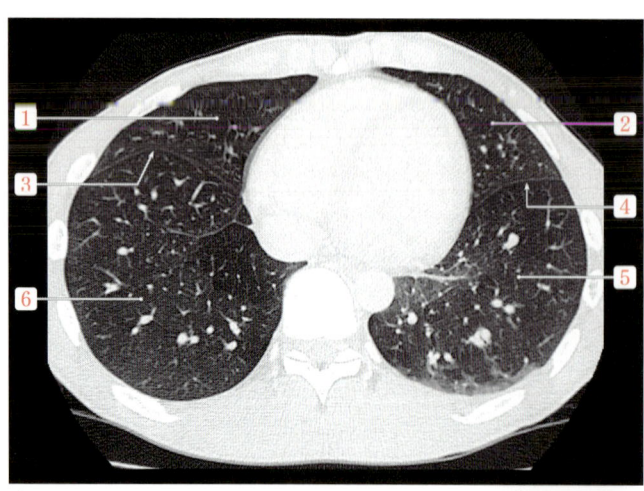

高分解能CT（肺野条件、横断像）

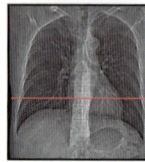

1 右肺中葉　Middle lobe of right lung
2 左肺上葉舌区　Lingular segment
3 右大葉間裂　Right major fissure
4 左大葉間裂　Left major fissure
5 左肺下葉　Lower lobe of left lung
6 右肺下葉　Lower lobe of right lung

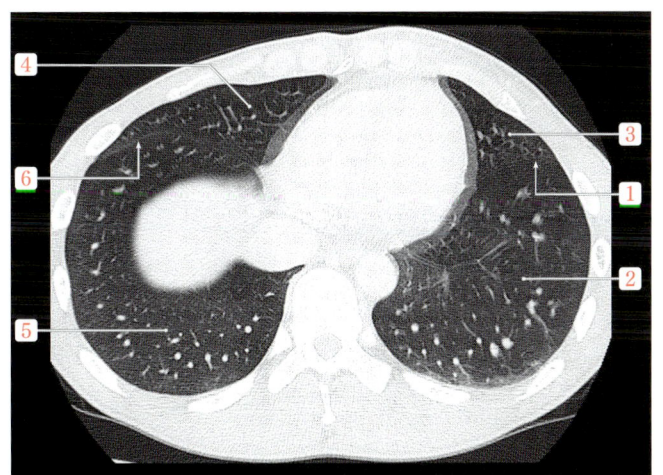

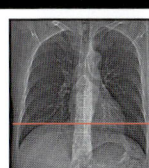

1　左大葉間裂　　Left major fissure
2　左肺下葉　　　Lower lobe of left lung
3　左肺上葉舌区　Lingular segment
4　右肺中葉　　　Middle lobe of right lung
5　右肺下葉　　　Lower lobe of right lung
6　右大葉間裂　　Right major fissure

高分解能CT（肺野条件、横断像）

胸部

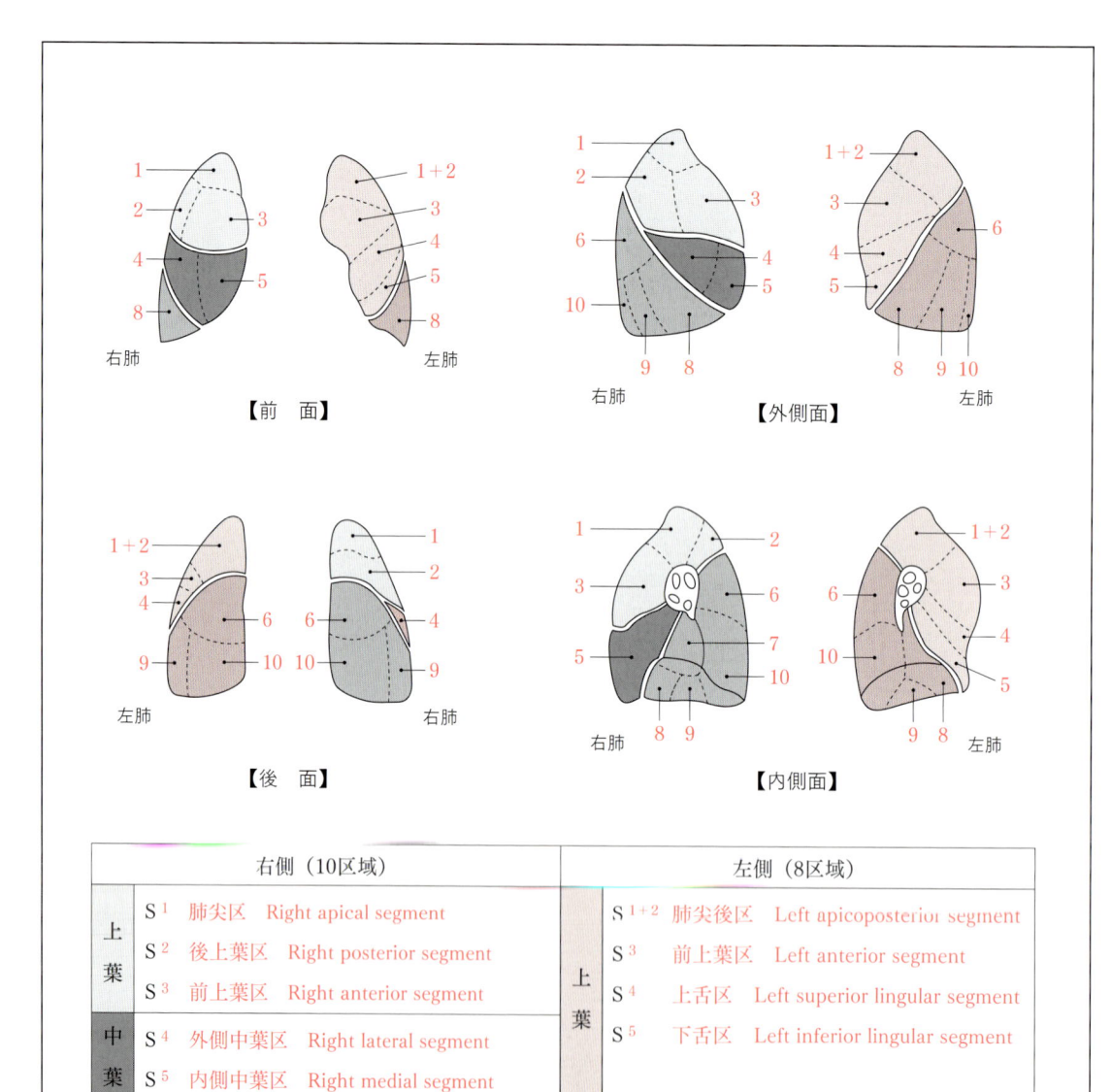

胸　部
Chest

【前　面】　右肺　左肺

【外側面】　右肺　左肺

【後　面】　左肺　右肺

【内側面】　右肺　左肺

	右側（10区域）			左側（8区域）		
上葉	S^1	肺尖区	Right apical segment	S^{1+2}	肺尖後区	Left apicoposterior segment
	S^2	後上葉区	Right posterior segment	S^3	前上葉区	Left anterior segment
	S^3	前上葉区	Right anterior segment			
中葉	S^4	外側中葉区	Right lateral segment	上葉	S^4	上舌区	Left superior lingular segment
	S^5	内側中葉区	Right medial segment		S^5	下舌区	Left inferior lingular segment
下葉	S^6	上-下葉区	Right superior segment	下葉	S^6	上-下葉区	Left superior segment
	S^7	内側肺底区	Right medial basal segment				
	S^8	前肺底区	Right anterior basal segment		S^8	前肺底区	Left anterior basal segment
	S^9	外側肺底区	Right lateral basal segment		S^9	外側肺底区	Left lateral basal segment
	S^{10}	後肺底区	Right posterior basal segment		S^{10}	後肺底区	Left posterior basal segment

参考図5　肺区域とその名称

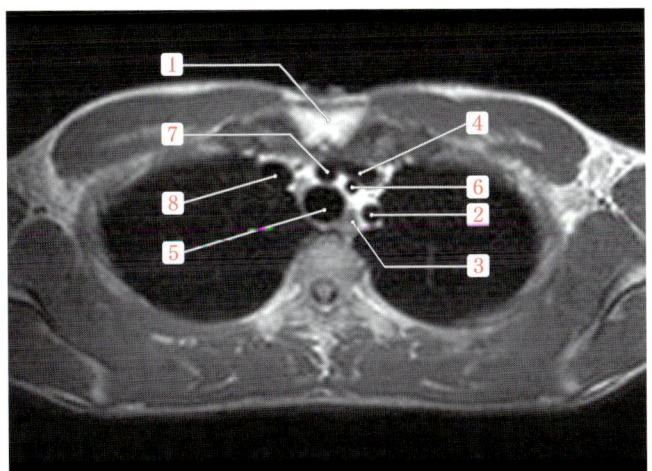

MRI T1強調像（横断像）

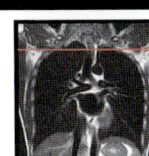

1　胸骨　　　　Sternum
2　左鎖骨下動脈　Left subclavian artery
3　食道　　　　Esophagus
4　左腕頭静脈　Left brachiocephalic vein
5　気管　　　　Trachea
6　左総頸動脈　Left common carotid artery
7　腕頭動脈　　Brachiocephalic artery
8　右腕頭静脈　Right brachiocephalic vein

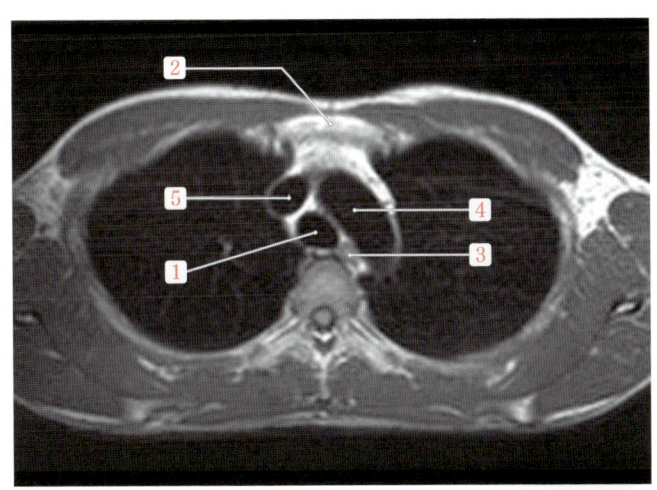

MRI T1強調像（横断像）

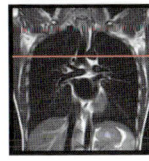

1　気管　　　Trachea
2　胸骨　　　Sternum
3　食道　　　Esophagus
4　大動脈弓　Aortic arch
5　上大静脈　Superior vena cava

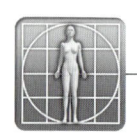

胸部
Chest

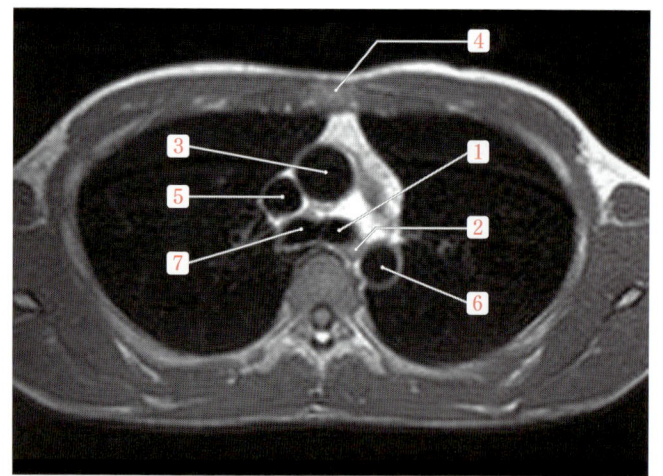

MRI T1強調像（横断像）

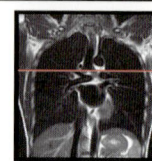

1 左主気管支　Left main bronchus
2 食道　Esophagus
3 上行大動脈　Ascending aorta
4 胸骨　Sternum
5 上大静脈　Superior vena cava
6 下行大動脈　Descending aorta
7 右主気管支　Right main bronchus

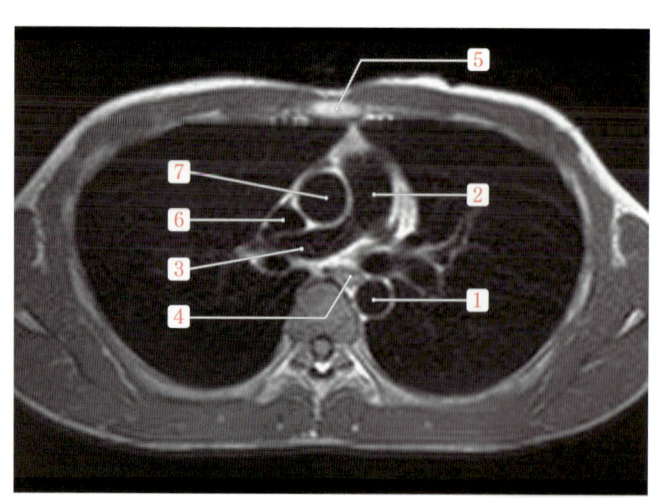

MRI T1強調像（横断像）

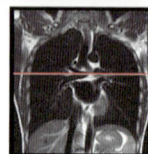

1 下行大動脈　Descending aorta
2 肺動脈幹　Pulmonary trunk
3 右肺動脈　Right pulmonary artery
4 食道　Esophagus
5 胸骨　Sternum
6 上大静脈　Superior vena cava
7 上行大動脈　Ascending aorta

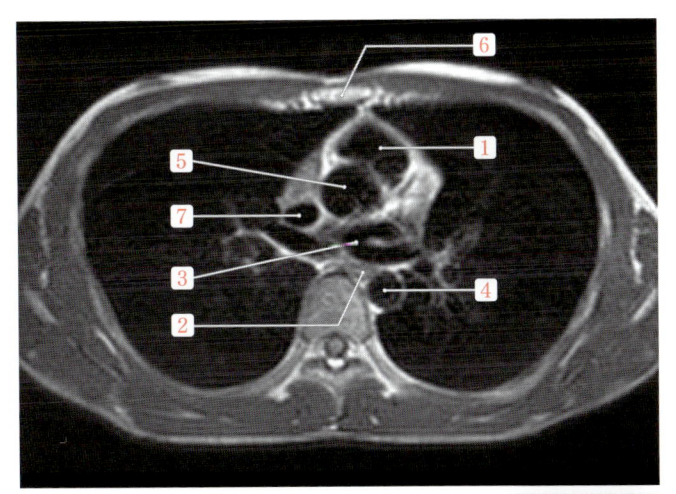

MRI T1強調像（横断像）

1 肺動脈弁　Pulmonary valve
2 食道　Esophagus
3 左心房　Left atrium
4 下行大動脈　Descending aorta
5 大動脈弁　Aortic valve
6 胸骨　Sternum
7 上大静脈　Superior vena cava

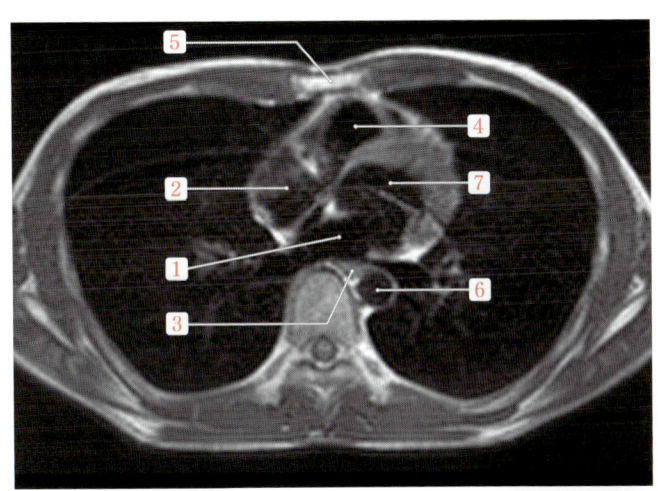

MRI T1強調像（横断像）

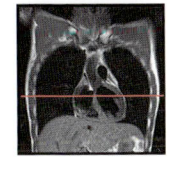

1 左心房　Left atrium
2 右心房　Right atrium
3 食道　Esophagus
4 右心室　Right ventricle
5 胸骨　Sternum
6 下行大動脈　Descending aorta
7 左心室　Left ventricle

胸部

61

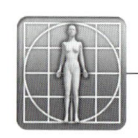

胸部
Chest

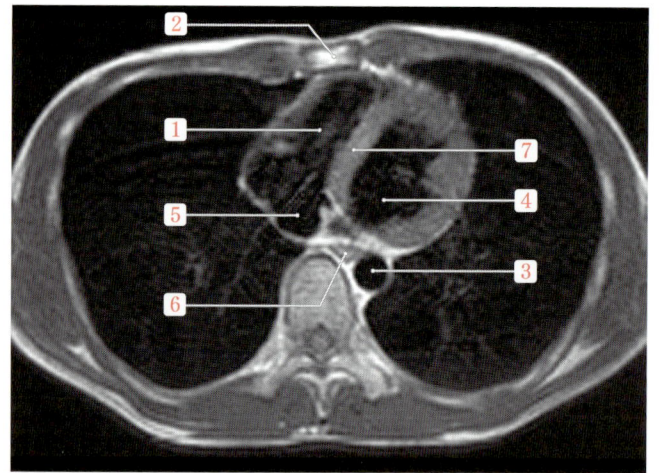

MRI T1 強調像（横断像）

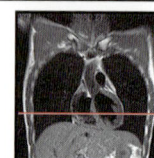

1 右心室　Right ventricle
2 胸骨　Sternum
3 下行大動脈　Descending aorta
4 左心室　Left ventricle
5 下大静脈　Inferior vena cava
6 食道　Esophagus
7 心室中隔　Interventricular septum

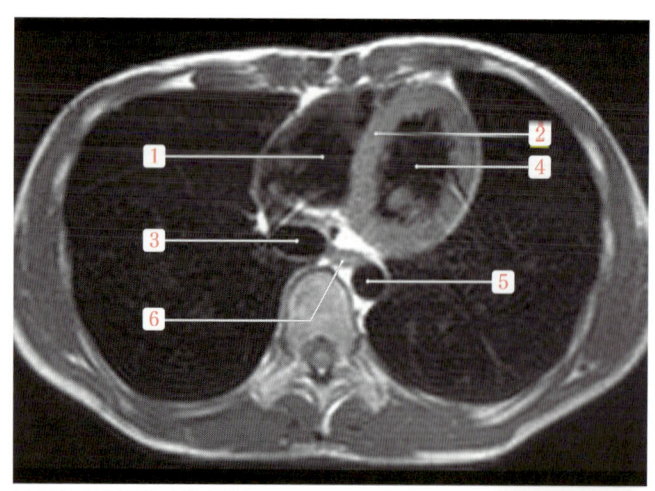

MRI T1 強調像（横断像）

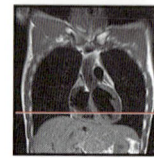

1 右心室　Right ventricle
2 心室中隔　Interventricular septum
3 下大静脈　Inferior vena cava
4 左心室　Left ventricle
5 下行大動脈　Descending aorta
6 食道　Esophagus

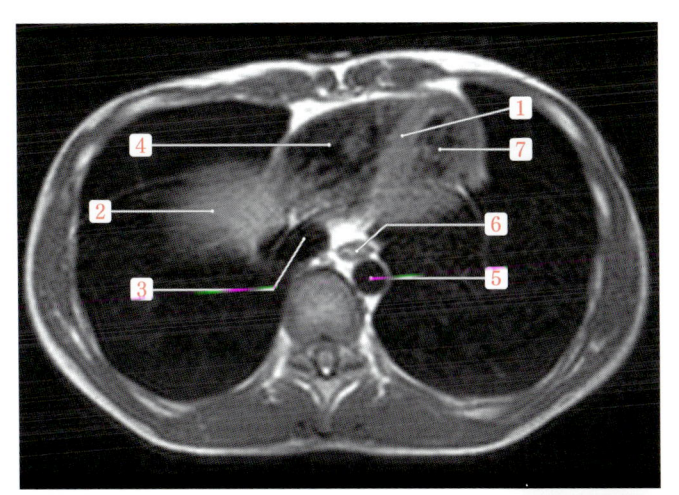

MRI T1強調像（横断像）

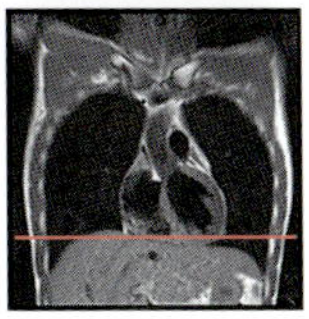

1 心室中隔　Interventricular septum
2 肝臓　Liver
3 下大静脈　Inferior vena cava
4 右心室　Right ventricle
5 下行大動脈　Descending aorta
6 食道　Esophagus
7 左心室　Left ventricle

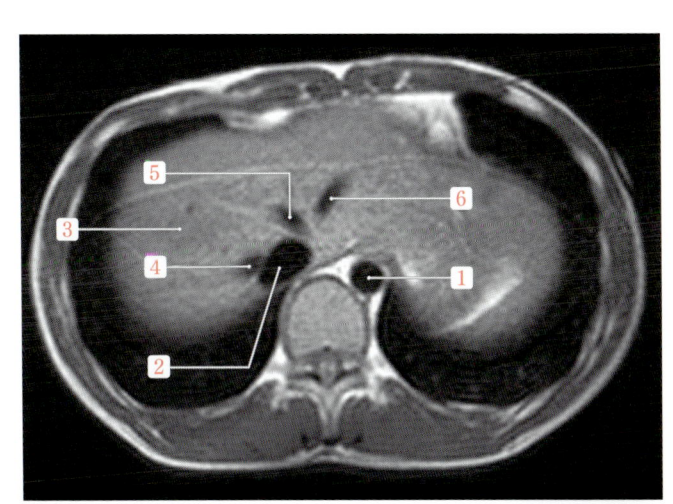

MRI T1強調像（横断像）

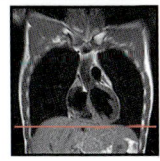

1 下行大動脈　Descending aorta
2 下大静脈　Inferior vena cava
3 肝臓　Liver
4 右肝静脈　Right hepatic vein
5 中肝静脈　Middle hepatic vein
6 左肝静脈　Left hepatic vein

63

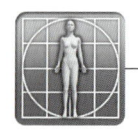

胸部
Chest

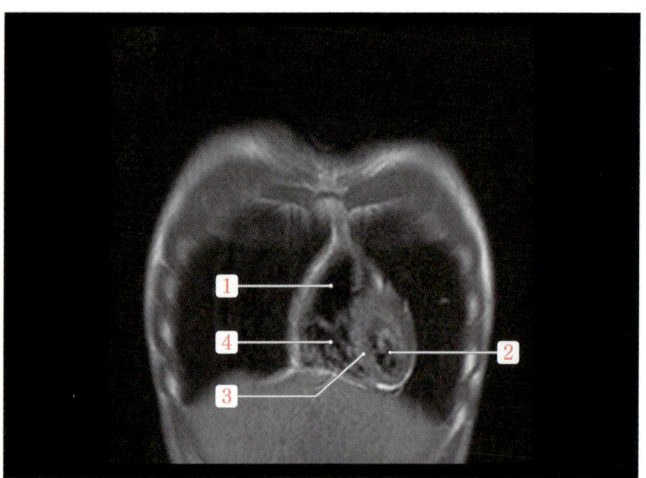

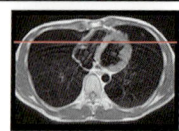

1 肺動脈幹　Pulmonary trunk
2 左心室　Left ventricle
3 心室中隔　Interventricular septum
4 右心室　Right ventricle

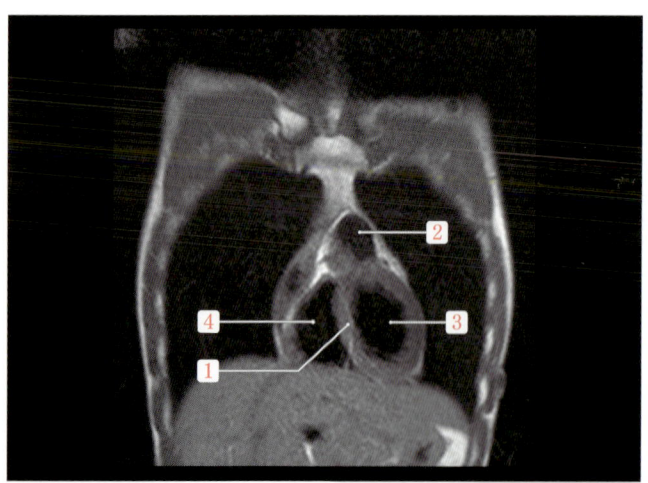

MRI T1強調像（冠状断像）

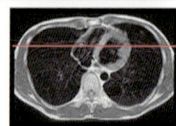

1 心室中隔　Interventricular septum
2 肺動脈幹　Pulmonary trunk
3 左心室　Left ventricle
4 右心室　Right ventricle

MRI T1強調像（冠状断像）

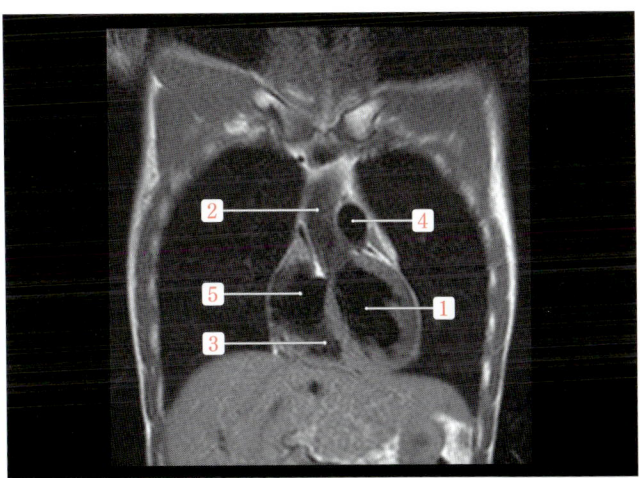

MRI T1強調像（冠状断像）

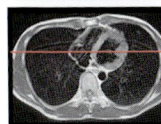

1 左心室　Left ventricle
2 上行大動脈　Ascending aorta
3 右心室　Right ventricle
4 肺動脈幹　Pulmonary trunk
5 右心房　Right atrium

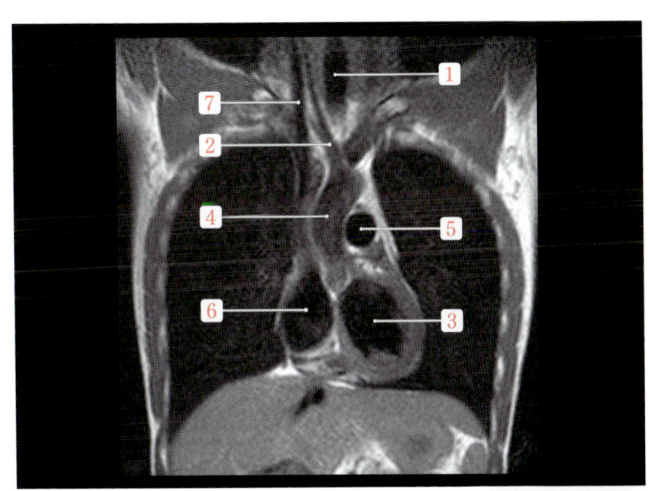

MRI T1強調像（冠状断像）

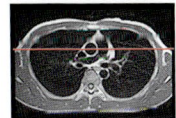

1 気管　Trachea
2 腕頭動脈　Brachiocephalic artery
3 左心室　Left ventricle
4 上行大動脈　Ascending aorta
5 肺動脈幹　Pulmonary trunk
6 右心房　Right atrium
7 右腕頭静脈　Right brachiocephalic vein

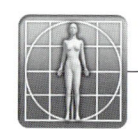

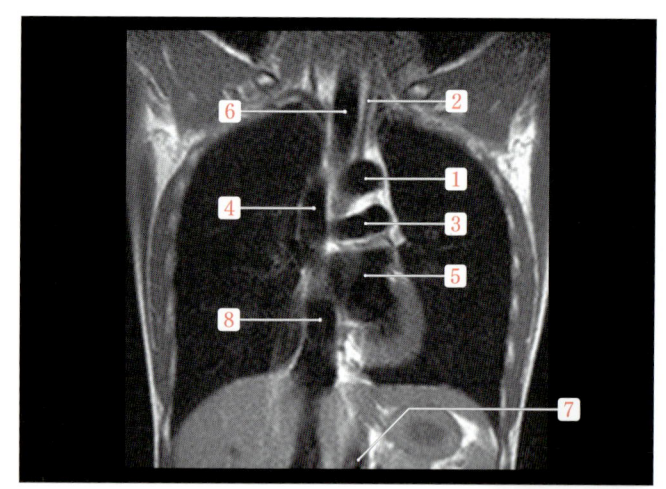

胸部
Chest

MRI T1強調像（冠状断像）

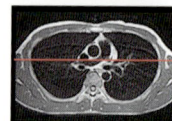

1 大動脈弓　Aortic arch
2 左総頸動脈　Left common carotid artery
3 肺動脈　Pulmonary artery
4 上大静脈　Superior vena cava
5 左心房　Left atrium
6 気管　Trachea
7 腹部大動脈　Abdominal aorta
8 下大静脈　Inferior vena cava

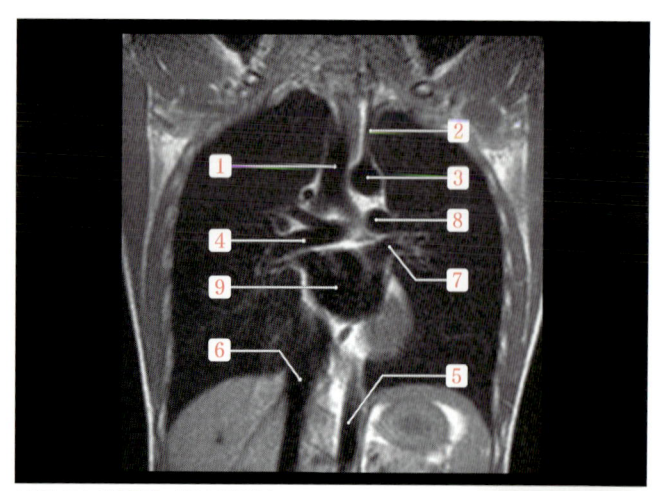

MRI T1強調像（冠状断像）

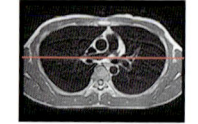

1 気管　Trachea
2 左鎖骨下動脈　Left subclavian artery
3 大動脈弓　Aortic arch
4 右肺動脈　Right pulmonary artery
5 腹部大動脈　Abdominal aorta
6 下大静脈　Inferior vena cava
7 左肺静脈　Left pulmonary vein
8 左肺動脈　Left pulmonary artery
9 左心房　Left atrium

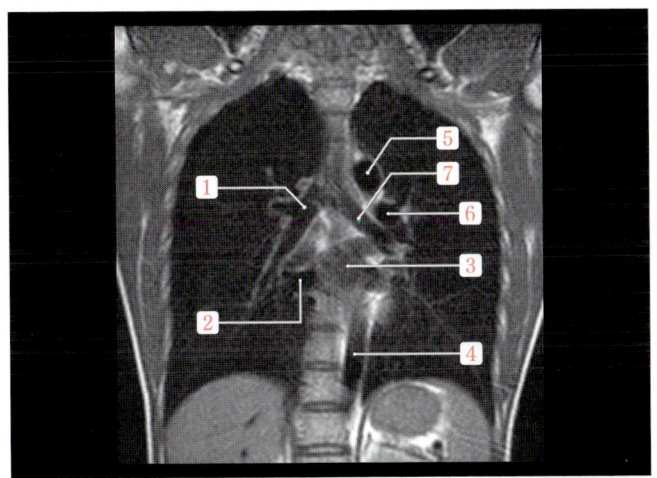

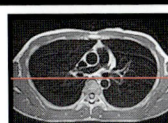

1　右主気管支　Right main bronchus
2　右肺静脈　Right pulmonary vein
3　左心房　Left atrium
4　下行大動脈　Descending aorta
5　大動脈弓　Aortic arch
6　左肺動脈　Left pulmonary artery
7　左主気管支　Left main bronchus

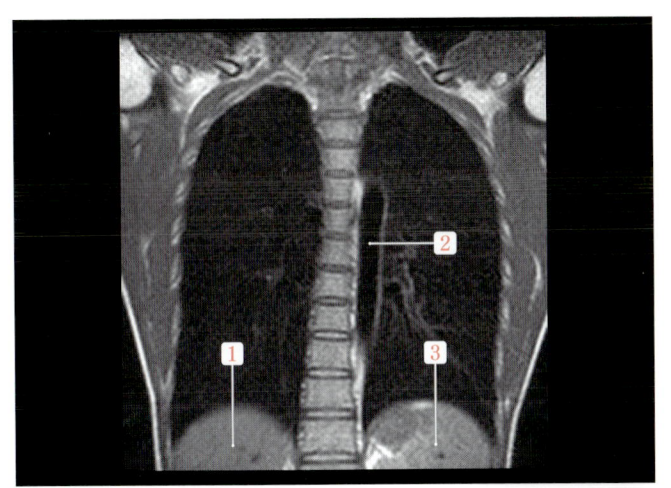

MRI T1強調像（冠状断像）

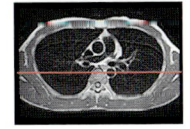

1　肝臓　Liver
2　下行大動脈　Descending aorta
3　脾臓　Spleen

MRI T1強調像（冠状断像）

胸部

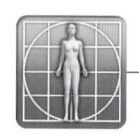

| 胸 部
| Chest

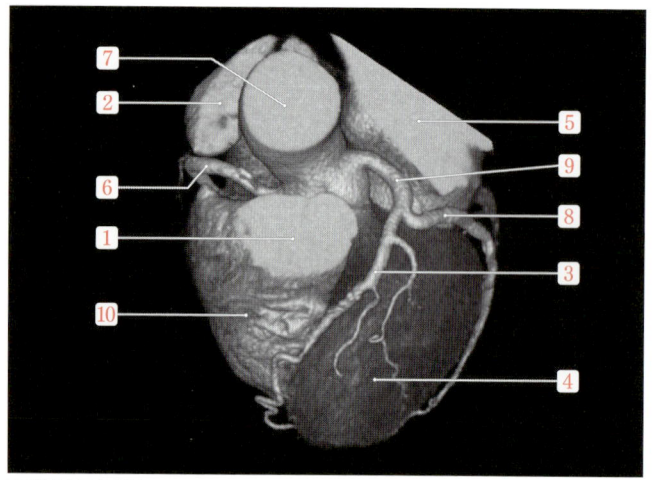

冠動脈 3DCT

1 肺動脈幹　Pulmonary trunk
2 右心耳　Right auricle
3 左冠動脈前下行枝 (LAD)
　Left anterior descending coronary artery
4 左心室　Left ventricle
5 左心房　Left atrium
6 右冠動脈 (RCA)　Right coronary artery
7 上行大動脈　Ascending aorta
8 左冠動脈回旋枝 (LCX)
　Left circumflex coronary artery
9 左冠動脈主幹部 (LMT)
　Left coronary artery main stem
10 右心室　Right ventricle

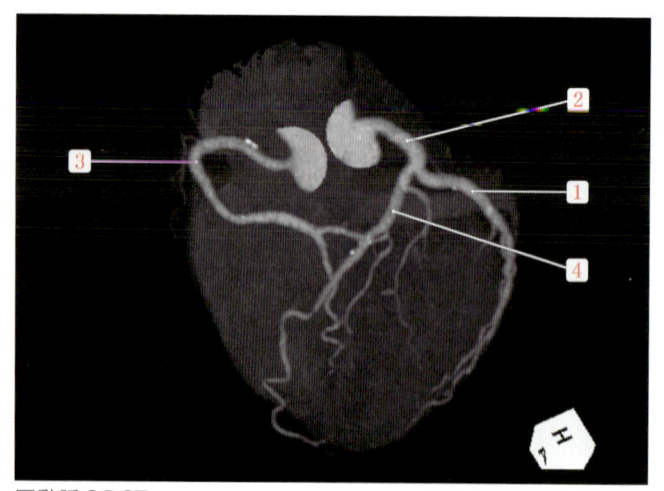

冠動脈 3DCT

1 左冠動脈回旋枝 (LCX)
　Left circumflex coronary artery
2 左冠動脈主幹部 (LMT)
　Left coronary artery main stem
3 右冠動脈 (RCA)　Right coronary artery
4 左冠動脈前下行枝 (LAD)
　Left anterior descending coronary artery

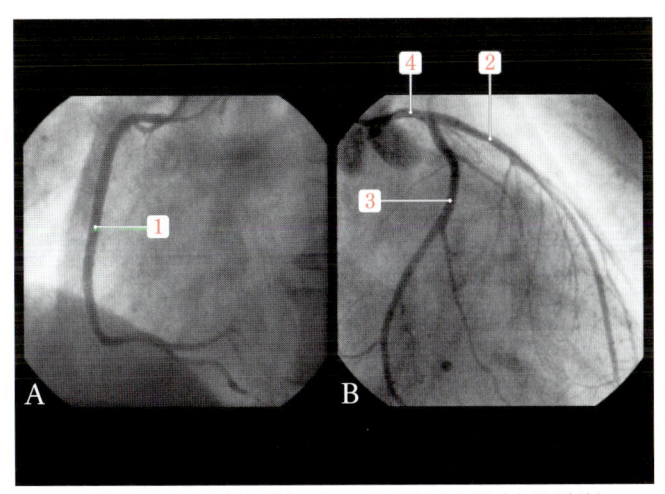

1 右冠動脈（RCA）　Right coronary artery
2 左冠動脈前下行枝（LAD）
　Left anterior descending coronary artery
3 左冠動脈回旋枝（LCX）
　Left circumflex coronary artery
4 左冠動脈主幹部（LMT）
　Left coronary artcry main stem

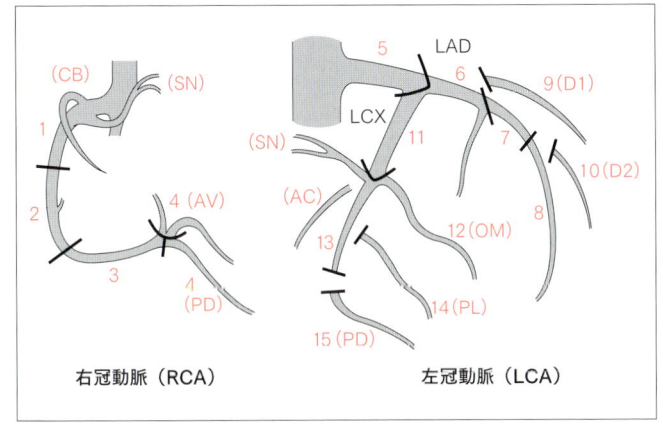

A：右冠動脈造影（左前斜位）、B：左冠動脈造影（右前斜位）

RCA（右冠動脈 Right coronary artery）
CB（円錐枝 Conus branch）
SN（洞結節動脈 Sinus node artery）
AV（房室枝 A-V node artery）
LCA（左冠動脈 Left coronary artery）
LAD（左冠動脈前下行枝 Left anterior descending coronary artery）
D1（第1対角枝 First diagonal branch）
D2（第2対角枝 Second diagonal branch）
LCX（左冠動脈回旋枝 Left circumflex coronary artery）
OM（鈍縁枝 Obtuse marginal branch）
AC（心房回旋枝 Atrial circumflex branch）
PL（後側壁枝 Posterolateral branch）
PD（後下行枝 Posterior descending branch）

参考図6　アメリカ心臓協会（AHA）による冠動脈セグメント

【右冠動脈（RCA）】
　起始部より右室下壁に鋭角に屈曲している部分までを2等分し、近位部を1、遠位部を2とする。それより後下行枝（PD）までが3、後下行枝と3より末梢を4とする。

【左冠動脈（LCA）】
　主幹部は5、前下行枝起始部から大きな第1中隔枝までは6、前下行枝末端までを2等分し、7、8とする。9、10は左室側面方向に分布する対角枝であり、第1対角枝を9、第2対角枝を10とする。回旋枝は鈍縁枝までを11、鈍縁枝を12、鈍縁枝より末梢の回旋枝を13とする。また、後側壁枝は14、後下行枝が回旋枝より分岐する場合は15とする。

胸 部
Chest

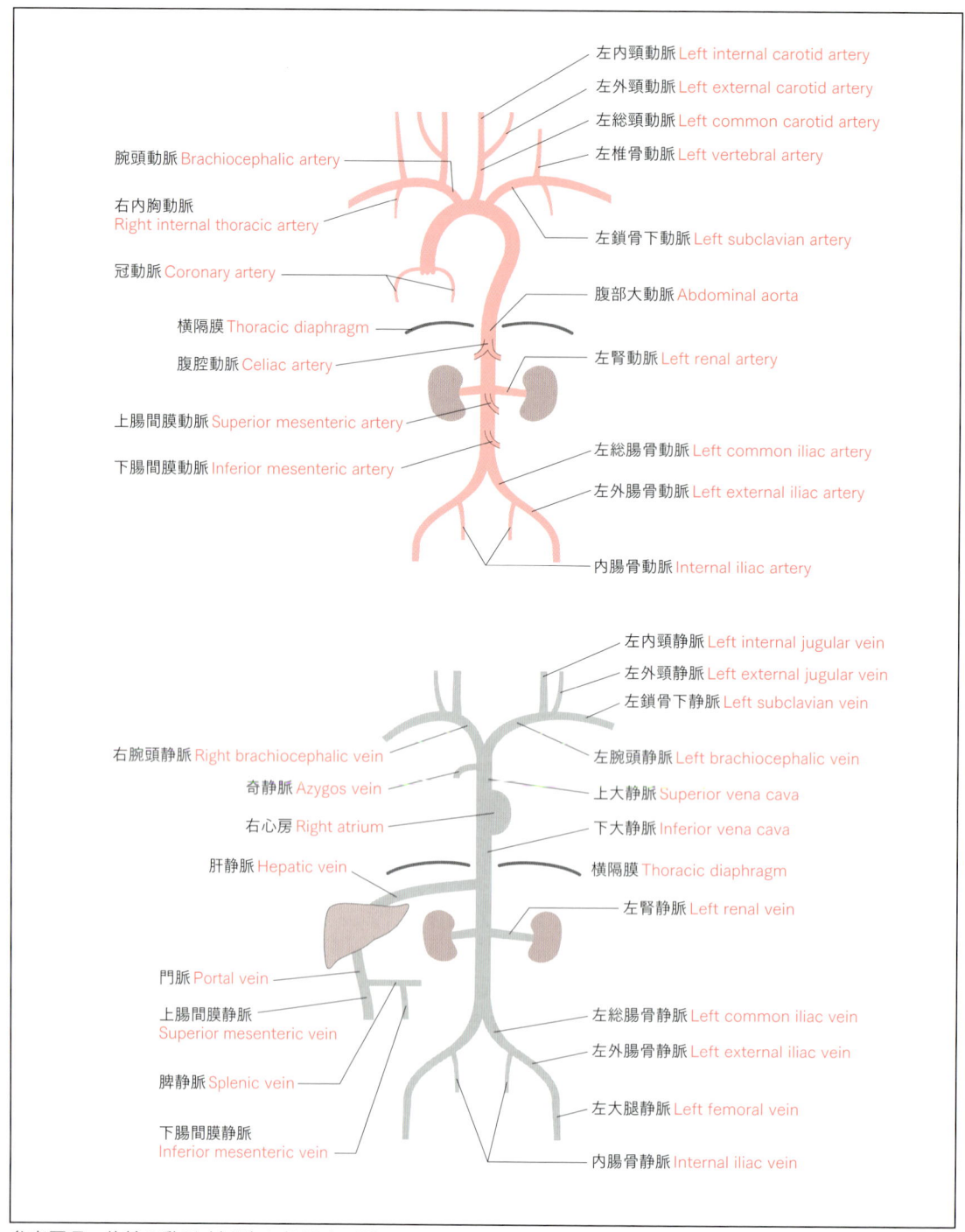

左内頸動脈 Left internal carotid artery
左外頸動脈 Left external carotid artery
左総頸動脈 Left common carotid artery
左椎骨動脈 Left vertebral artery
腕頭動脈 Brachiocephalic artery
右内胸動脈 Right internal thoracic artery
左鎖骨下動脈 Left subclavian artery
冠動脈 Coronary artery
腹部大動脈 Abdominal aorta
横隔膜 Thoracic diaphragm
腹腔動脈 Celiac artery
左腎動脈 Left renal artery
上腸間膜動脈 Superior mesenteric artery
下腸間膜動脈 Inferior mesenteric artery
左総腸骨動脈 Left common iliac artery
左外腸骨動脈 Left external iliac artery
内腸骨動脈 Internal iliac artery

左内頸静脈 Left internal jugular vein
左外頸静脈 Left external jugular vein
左鎖骨下静脈 Left subclavian vein
右腕頭静脈 Right brachiocephalic vein
奇静脈 Azygos vein
左腕頭静脈 Left brachiocephalic vein
上大静脈 Superior vena cava
右心房 Right atrium
下大静脈 Inferior vena cava
肝静脈 Hepatic vein
横隔膜 Thoracic diaphragm
左腎静脈 Left renal vein
門脈 Portal vein
上腸間膜静脈 Superior mesenteric vein
左総腸骨静脈 Left common iliac vein
脾静脈 Splenic vein
左外腸骨静脈 Left external iliac vein
左大腿静脈 Left femoral vein
下腸間膜静脈 Inferior mesenteric vein
内腸骨静脈 Internal iliac vein

参考図7　体幹の動脈（上段）と静脈（下段）（アイメディスン《iMedicine》1. 循環器. リブロ・サイエンス, 2008, p.21・23 より）

CT・MRI 解体新書

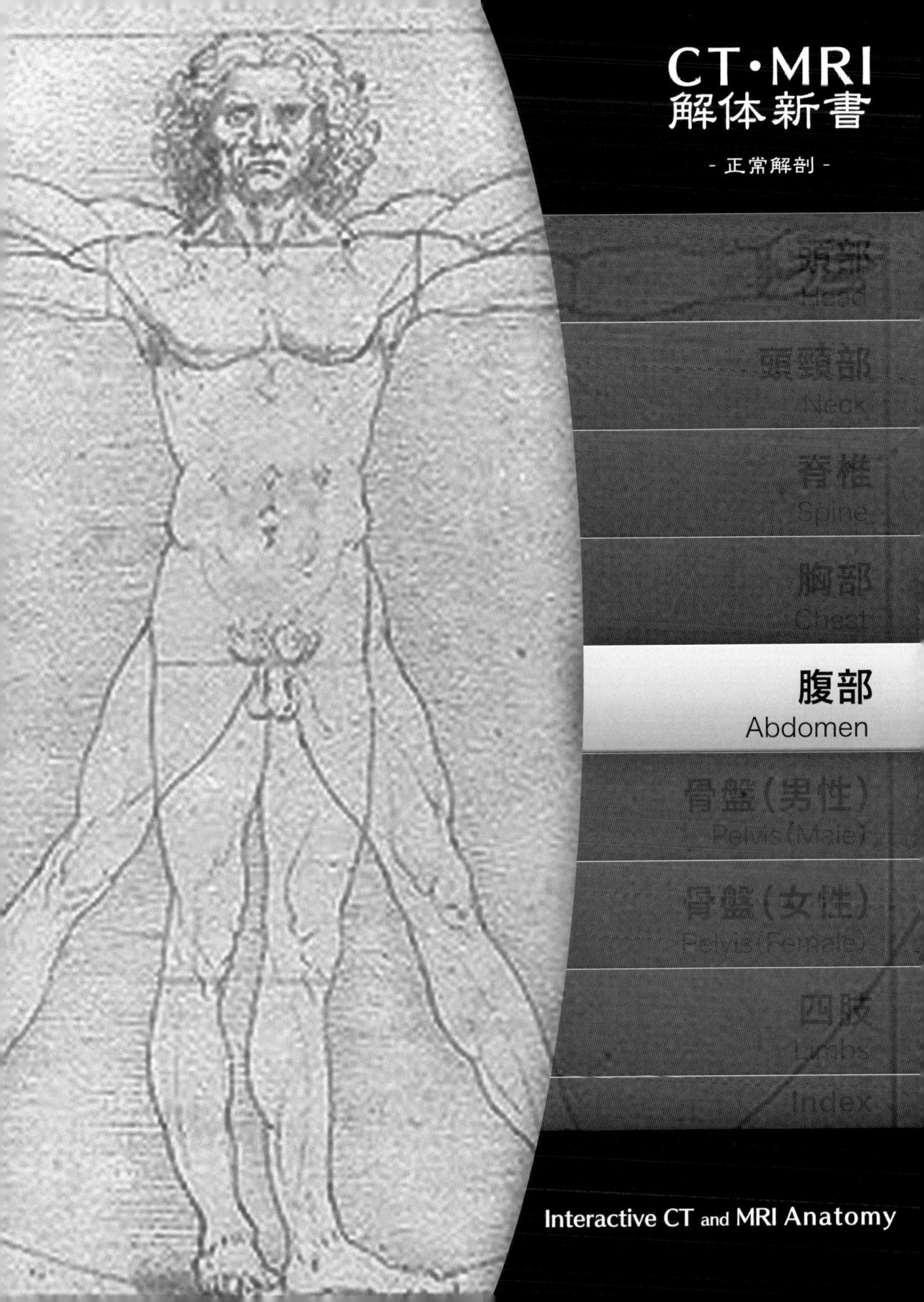

- 正常解剖 -

頭部 Head

頭頸部 Neck

脊椎 Spine

胸部 Chest

腹部
Abdomen

骨盤(男性) Pelvis (Male)

骨盤(女性) Pelvis (Female)

四肢 Limbs

Index

Interactive CT and MRI Anatomy

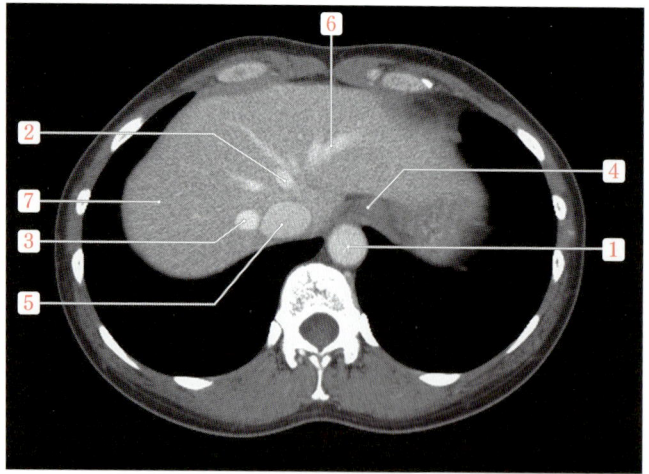

腹 部
Abdomen

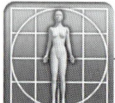

造影CT（横断像）

1 下行大動脈　Descending aorta
2 中肝静脈　Middle hepatic vein
3 右肝静脈　Right hepatic vein
4 食道胃移行部　Esophagogastric junction
5 下大静脈　Inferior vena cava
6 左肝静脈　Left hepatic vein
7 肝臓　Liver

造影CT（横断像）

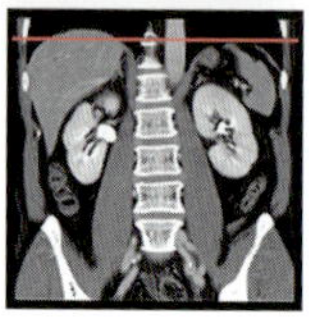

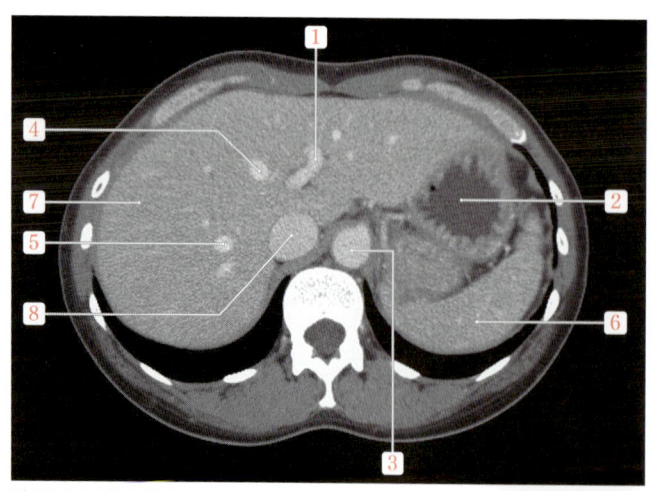

1 門脈左枝　Left portal vein
2 胃　Stomach
3 腹部大動脈　Abdominal aorta
4 中肝静脈　Middle hepatic vein
5 右肝静脈　Right hepatic vein
6 脾臓　Spleen
7 肝臓　Liver
8 下大静脈　Inferior vena cava

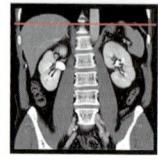

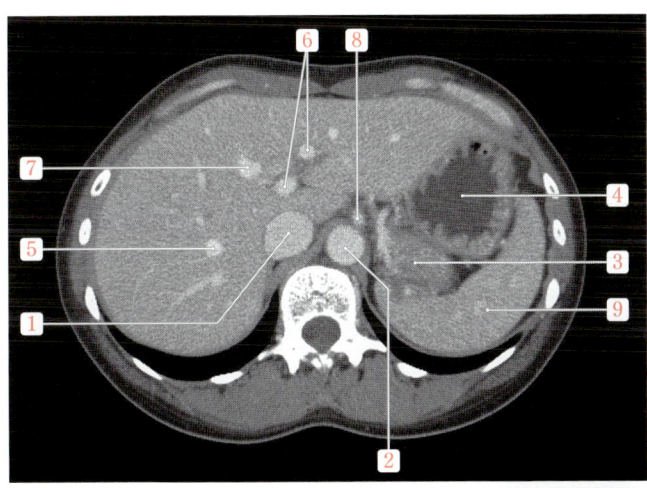

造影CT（横断像）

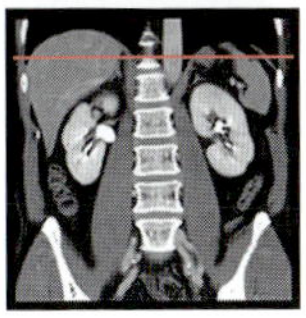

1 下大静脈　Inferior vena cava
2 腹部大動脈　Abdominal aorta
3 膵臓　Pancreas
4 胃　Stomach
5 右肝静脈　Right hepatic vein
6 門脈左枝　Left portal vein
7 中肝静脈　Middle hepatic vein
8 腹腔動脈　Celiac artery
9 脾臓　Spleen

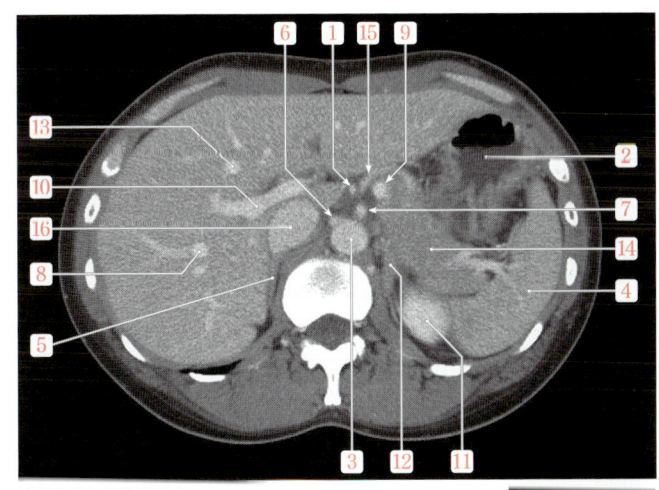

造影CT（横断像）

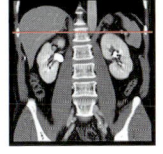

1 総肝動脈　Common hepatic artery
2 胃　Stomach
3 腹部大動脈　Abdominal aorta
4 脾臓　Spleen
5 右副腎　Right adrenal gland
6 右腎動脈　Right renal artery
7 腹腔動脈　Celiac artery
8 右肝静脈　Right hepatic vein
9 脾静脈　Splenic vein
10 門脈右枝　Right portal vein
11 左腎　Left kidney
12 左副腎　Left adrenal gland
13 中肝静脈　Middle hepatic vein
14 膵臓　Pancreas
15 脾動脈　Splenic artery
16 下大静脈　Inferior vena cava

腹部
Abdomen

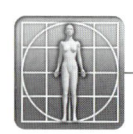

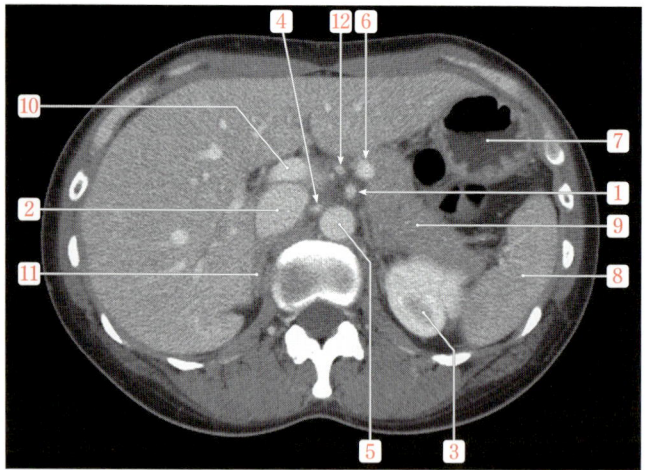

造影CT（横断像）

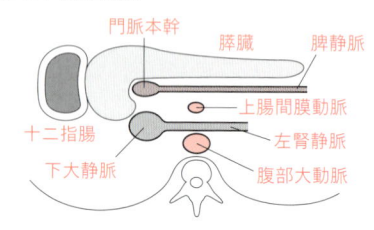

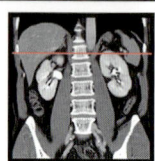

1 上腸間膜動脈　Superior mesenteric artery
2 下大静脈　Inferior vena cava
3 左腎　Left kidney
4 右腎動脈　Right renal artery
5 腹部大動脈　Abdominal aorta
6 脾静脈　Splenic vein
7 胃　Stomach
8 脾臓　Spleen
9 膵臓　Pancreas
10 門脈本幹　Main portal vein
11 右副腎　Right adrenal gland
12 総肝動脈　Common hepatic artery

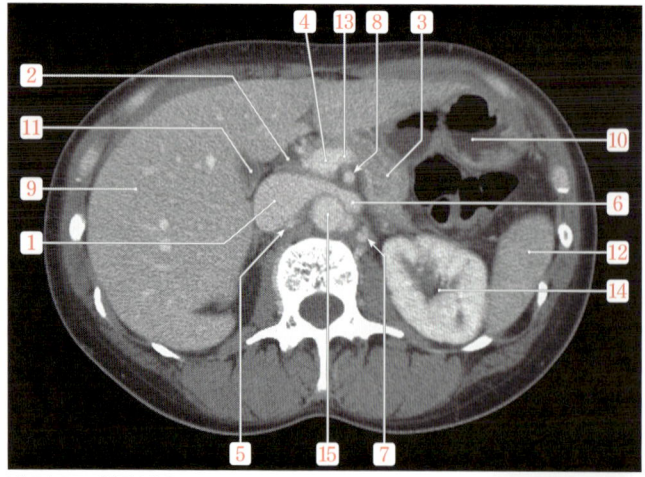

模式図：門脈本幹、膵臓、脾静脈、十二指腸、上腸間膜動脈、下大静脈、左腎静脈、腹部大動脈

造影CT（横断像）

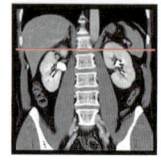

1 下大静脈　Inferior vena cava
2 総胆管　Common bile duct
3 膵臓　Pancreas
4 門脈本幹　Main portal vein
5 右腎動脈　Right renal artery
6 左腎静脈　Left renal vein
7 左腎動脈　Left renal artery
8 上腸間膜動脈　Superior mesenteric artery
9 肝臓　Liver
10 胃　Stomach
11 胆嚢　Gallbladder
12 脾臓　Spleen
13 脾静脈　Splenic vein
14 左腎　Left kidney
15 腹部大動脈　Abdominal aorta

74

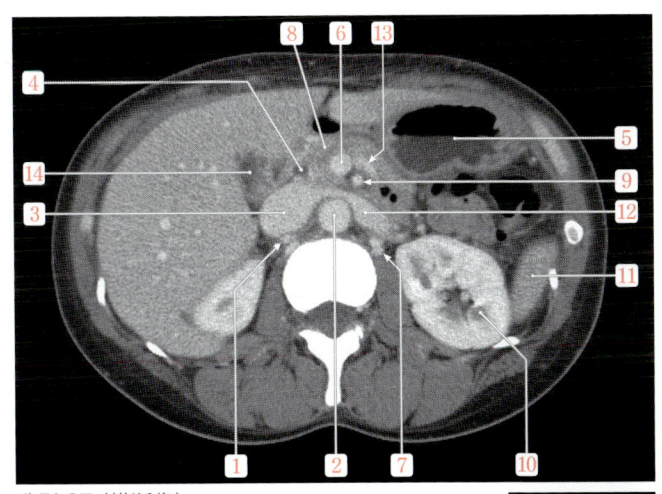

造影CT（横断像）

1 右腎動脈　Right renal artery
2 腹部大動脈　Abdominal aorta
3 下大静脈　Inferior vena cava
4 総胆管　Common bile duct
5 胃　Stomach
6 上腸間膜静脈　Superior mesenteric vein
7 左腎動脈　Left renal artery
8 膵臓　Pancreas
9 上腸間膜動脈
　Superior mesenteric artery
10 左腎　Left kidney
11 脾臓　Spleen
12 左腎静脈　Left renal vein
13 脾静脈　Splenic vein
14 胆嚢　Gallbladder

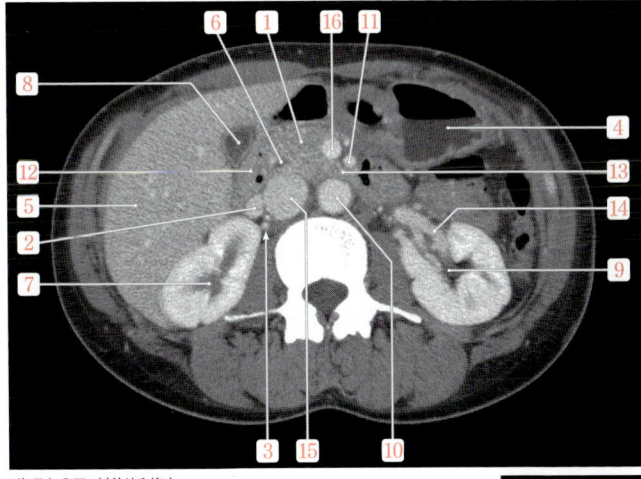

造影CT（横断像）

1 膵臓　Pancreas
2 右腎静脈　Right renal vein
3 右腎動脈　Right renal artery
4 胃　Stomach
5 肝臓　Liver
6 総胆管　Common bile duct
7 右腎　Right kidney
8 胆嚢　Gallbladder
9 左腎　Left kidney
10 腹部大動脈　Abdominal aorta
11 上腸間膜動脈
　Superior mesenteric artery
12 十二指腸　Duodenum
13 十二指腸水平脚
　Horizontal part of duodenum
14 左腎静脈　Left renal vein
15 下大静脈　Inferior vena cava
16 上腸間膜静脈　Superior mesenteric vein

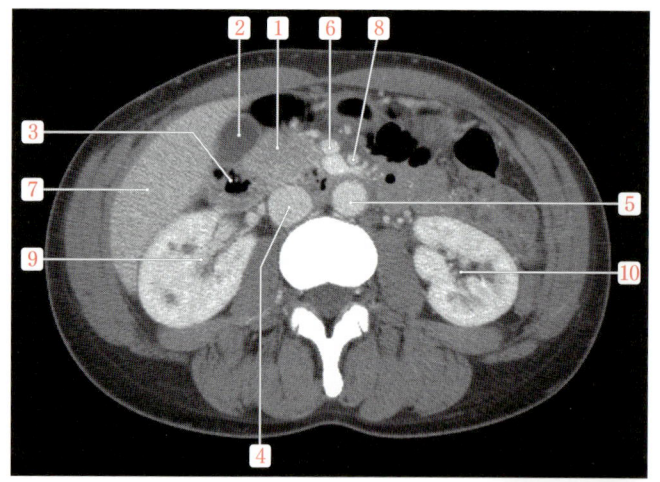

腹 部
Abdomen

造影CT（横断像）

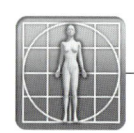

1 膵臓　Pancreas
2 胆嚢　Gallbladder
3 十二指腸　Duodenum
4 下大静脈　Inferior vena cava
5 腹部大動脈　Abdominal aorta
6 上腸間膜静脈　Superior mesenteric vein
7 肝臓　Liver
8 上腸間膜動脈　Superior mesenteric artery
9 右腎　Right kidney
10 左腎　Left kidney

造影CT（横断像）

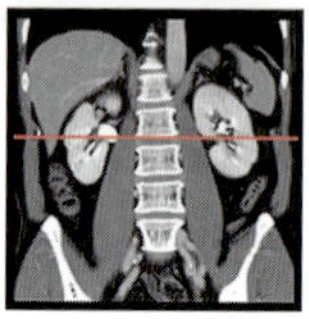

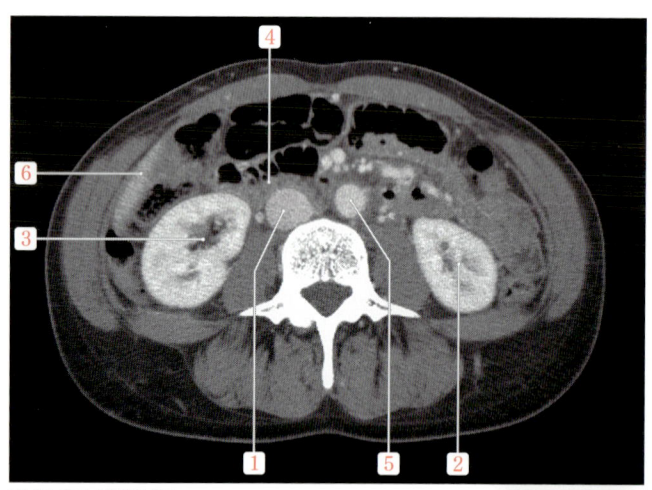

1 下大静脈　Inferior vena cava
2 左腎　Left kidney
3 右腎　Right kidney
4 十二指腸　Duodenum
5 腹部大動脈　Abdominal aorta
6 肝臓　Liver

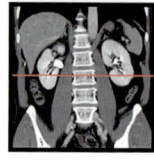

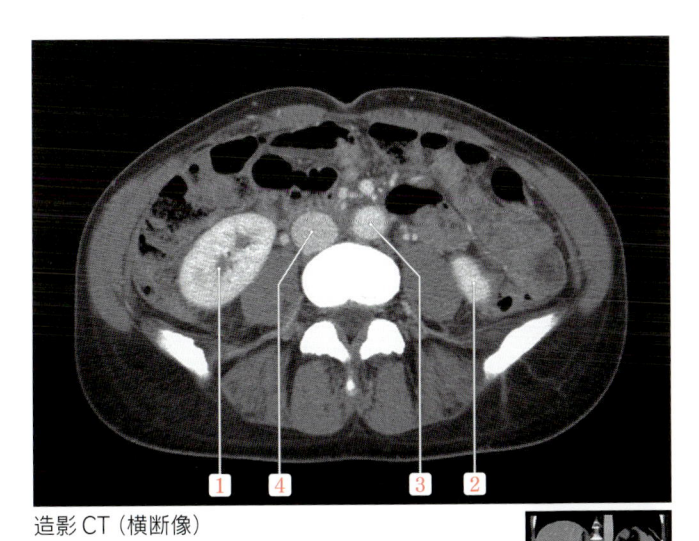

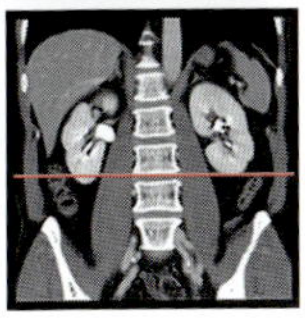

1　右腎　Right kidney
2　左腎　Left kidney
3　腹部大動脈　Abdominal aorta
4　下大静脈　Inferior vena cava

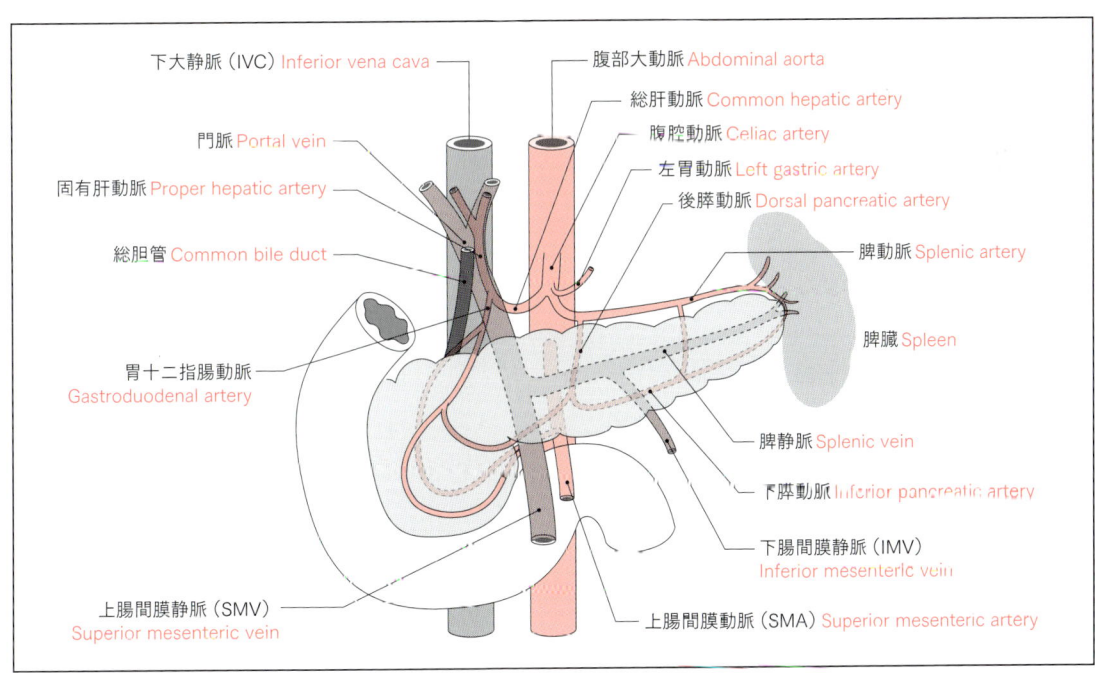

造影CT（横断像）

下大静脈（IVC）Inferior vena cava
腹部大動脈 Abdominal aorta
総肝動脈 Common hepatic artery
腹腔動脈 Celiac artery
門脈 Portal vein
左胃動脈 Left gastric artery
固有肝動脈 Proper hepatic artery
後膵動脈 Dorsal pancreatic artery
総胆管 Common bile duct
脾動脈 Splenic artery
脾臓 Spleen
胃十二指腸動脈 Gastroduodenal artery
脾静脈 Splenic vein
下膵動脈 Inferior pancreatic artery
下腸間膜静脈（IMV）Inferior mesenteric vein
上腸間膜静脈（SMV）Superior mesenteric vein
上腸間膜動脈（SMA）Superior mesenteric artery

参考図8　膵臓の脈管系

腹部
Abdomen

下大静脈
Inferior vena cava

胆囊 Gallbladder

Cantlie 線

【横隔面】　【臓側面】

下大静脈
Inferior vena cava

右肝静脈
Right hepatic vein

中肝静脈
Middle hepatic vein

左肝静脈
Left hepatic vein

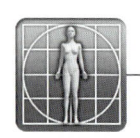

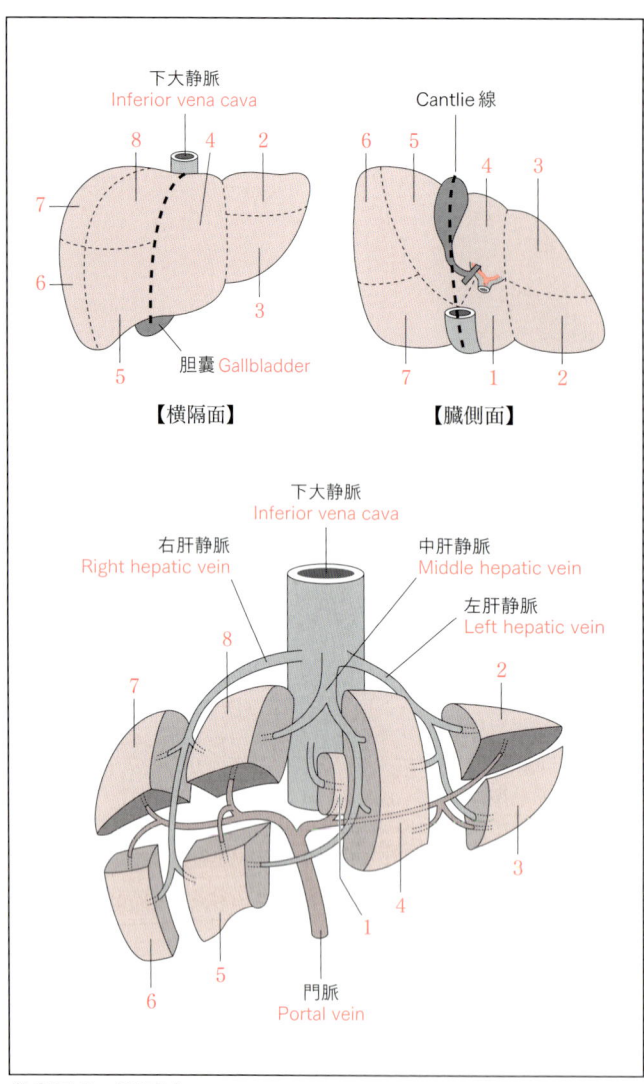

門脈
Portal vein

参考図9　肝区域

1　尾状葉
　　Caudate lobe
2　外側上区域
　　Left lateral superior segment
3　外側下区域
　　Left lateral inferior segment
4　内側区域
　　Left medial segment
5　前下区域
　　Right anterior inferior segment
6　後下区域
　　Right posterior inferior segment
7　後上区域
　　Right posterior superior segment
8　前上区域
　　Right anterior superior segment

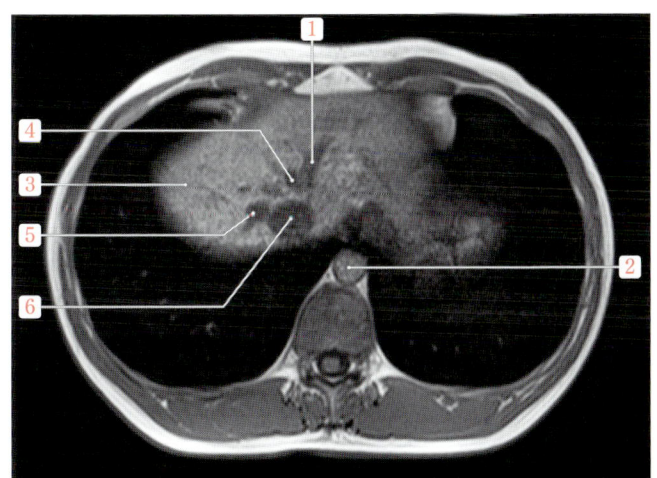

MRI T1強調像（横断像）

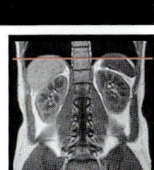

1 左肝静脈　Left hepatic vein
2 腹部大動脈　Abdominal aorta
3 肝臓　Liver
4 中肝静脈　Middle hepatic vein
5 右肝静脈　Right hepatic vein
6 下大静脈　Inferior vena cava

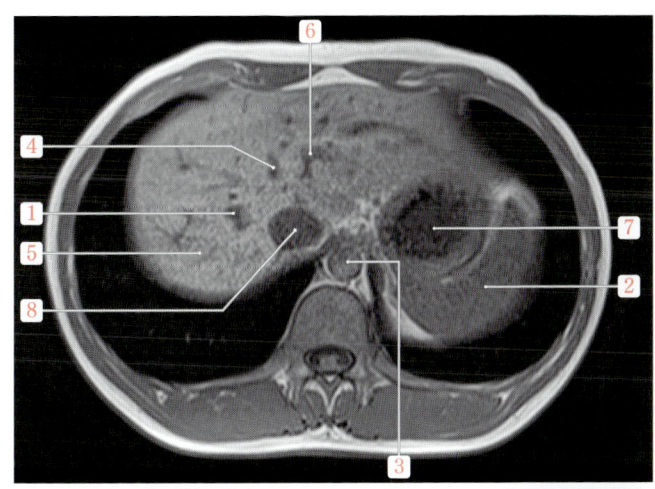

MRI T1強調像（横断像）

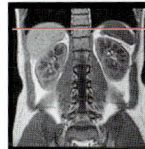

1 右肝静脈　Right hepatic vein
2 脾臓　Spleen
3 腹部大動脈　Abdominal aorta
4 中肝静脈　Middle hepatic vein
5 肝臓　Liver
6 左肝静脈　Left hepatic vein
7 胃　Stomach
8 下大静脈　Inferior vena cava

腹部
Abdomen

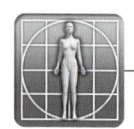

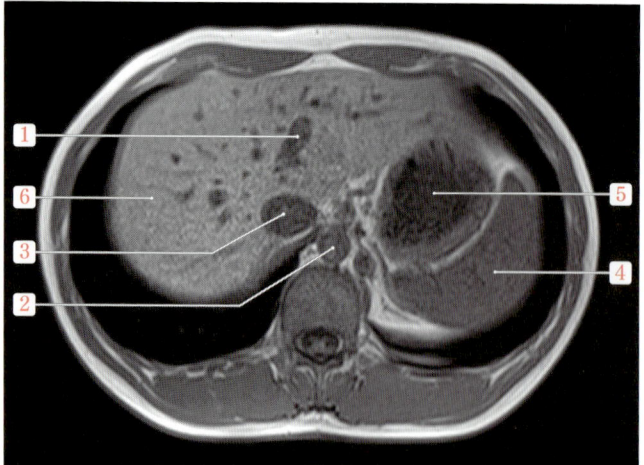

MRI T1強調像（横断像）

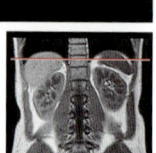

1 門脈左枝　Left portal vein
2 腹部大動脈　Abdominal aorta
3 下大静脈　Inferior vena cava
4 脾臓　Spleen
5 胃　Stomach
6 肝臓　Liver

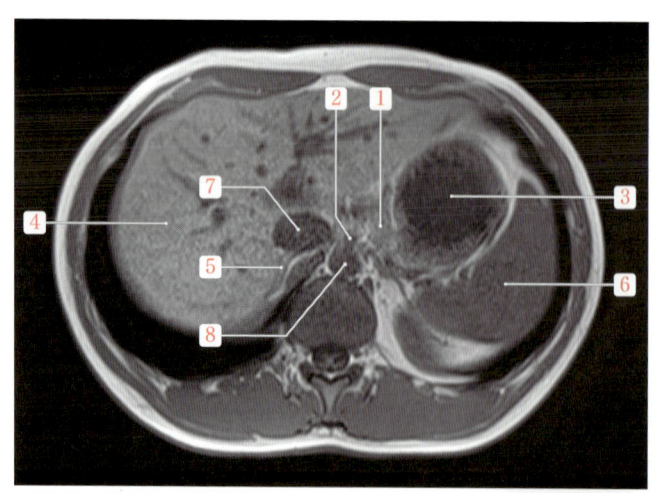

MRI T1強調像（横断像）

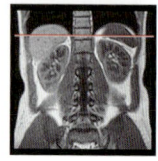

1 膵臓　Pancreas
2 腹腔動脈　Celiac artery
3 胃　Stomach
4 肝臓　Liver
5 右副腎　Right adrenal gland
6 脾臓　Spleen
7 下大静脈　Inferior vena cava
8 腹部大動脈　Abdominal aorta

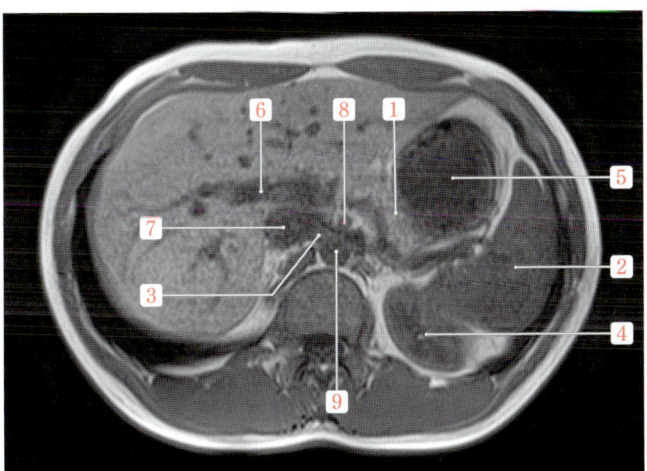

● CT・MRI 解体新書

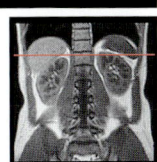

1　膵臓　Pancreas
2　脾臓　Spleen
3　左腎静脈　Left renal vein
4　左腎　Left kidney
5　胃　Stomach
6　門脈右枝　Right portal vein
7　下大静脈　Inferior vena cava
8　上腸間膜動脈
　　Superior mesenteric artery
9　腹部大動脈　Abdominal aorta

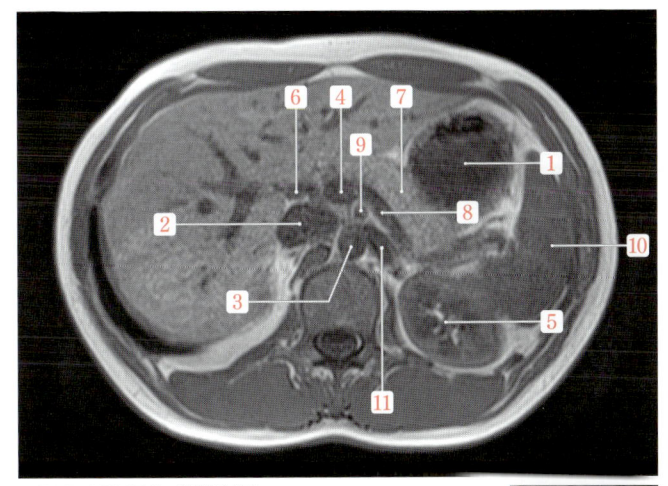

MRI T1強調像（横断像）

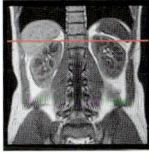

腹部

1　胃　Stomach
2　下大静脈　Inferior vena cava
3　腹部大動脈　Abdominal aorta
4　門脈本幹　Main portal vein
5　左腎　Left kidney
6　総胆管　Common bile duct
7　膵臓　Pancreas
8　脾静脈　Splenic vein
9　上腸間膜動脈
　　Superior mesenteric artery
10　脾臓　Spleen
11　左腎静脈　Left renal vein

MRI T1強調像（横断像）

81

腹 部
Abdomen

MRI T1強調像（横断像）

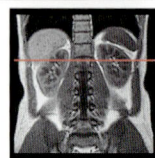

1 膵臓　Pancreas
2 左腎　Left kidney
3 右腎　Right kidney
4 胆嚢　Gallbladder
5 上腸間膜静脈　Superior mesenteric vein
6 腹部大動脈　Abdominal aorta
7 総胆管　Common bile duct
8 脾臓　Spleen
9 胃　Stomach
10 上腸間膜動脈　Superior mesenteric artery
11 下大静脈　Inferior vena cava

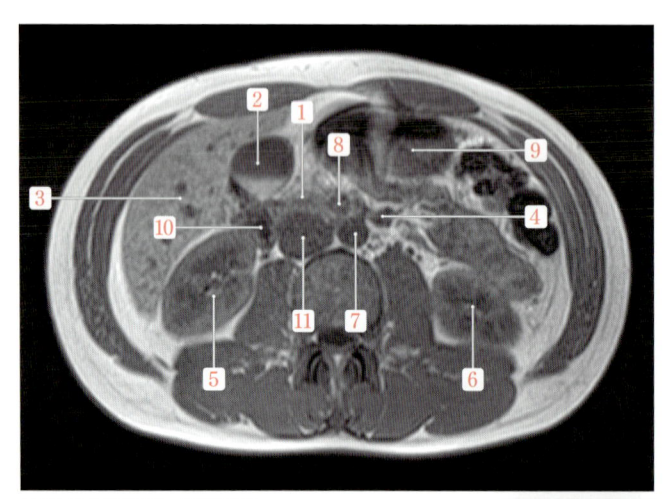

MRI T1強調像（横断像）

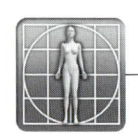

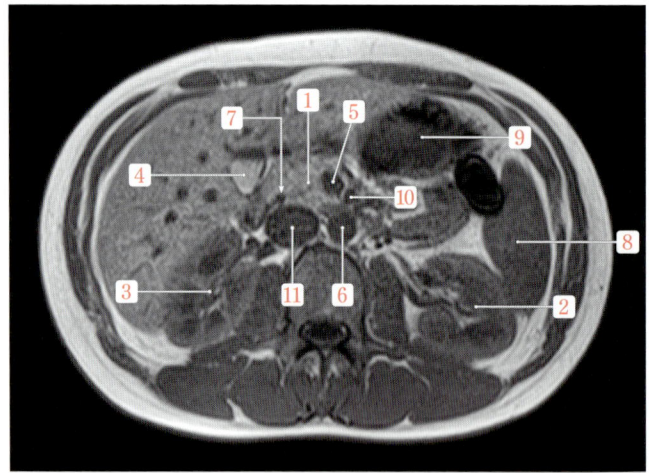

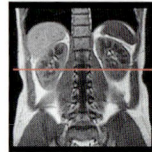

1 膵臓　Pancreas
2 胆嚢　Gallbladder
3 肝臓　Liver
4 上腸間膜動脈　Superior mesenteric artery
5 右腎　Right kidney
6 左腎　Left kidney
7 腹部大動脈　Abdominal aorta
8 上腸間膜静脈　Superior mesenteric vein
9 胃　Stomach
10 十二指腸　Duodenum
11 下大静脈　Inferior vena cava

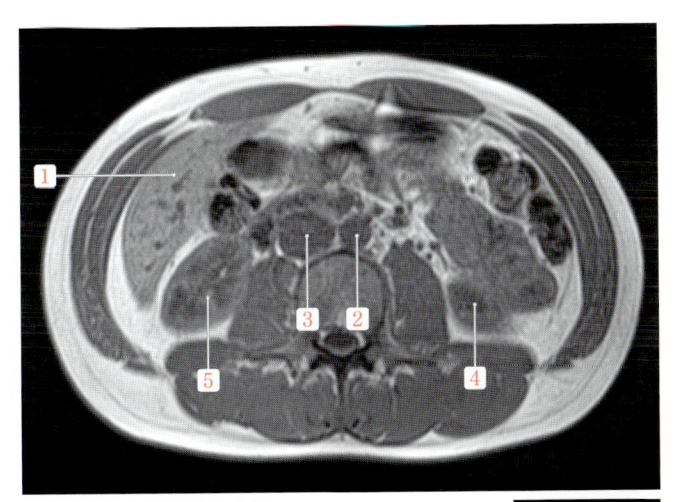

● CT・MRI 解体新書

1　肝臓　　Liver
2　腹部大動脈　Abdominal aorta
3　下大静脈　Inferior vena cava
4　左腎　　Left kidney
5　右腎　　Right kidney

MRI T1強調像（横断像）

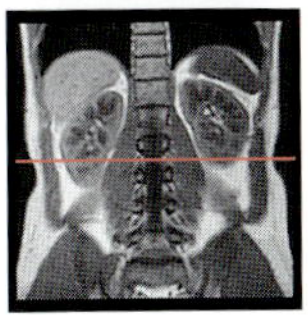

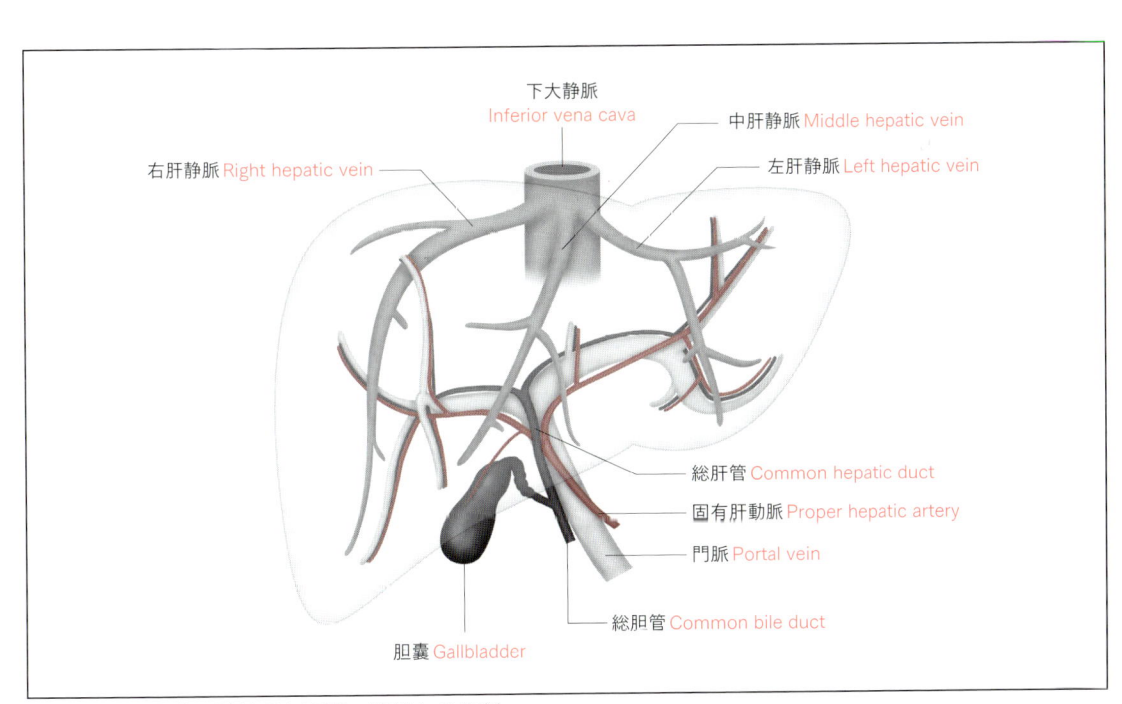

腹部

下大静脈 Inferior vena cava
中肝静脈 Middle hepatic vein
右肝静脈 Right hepatic vein
左肝静脈 Left hepatic vein
総肝管 Common hepatic duct
固有肝動脈 Proper hepatic artery
門脈 Portal vein
総胆管 Common bile duct
胆嚢 Gallbladder

参考図10　肝臓の脈管系と胆嚢・胆管との関係

83

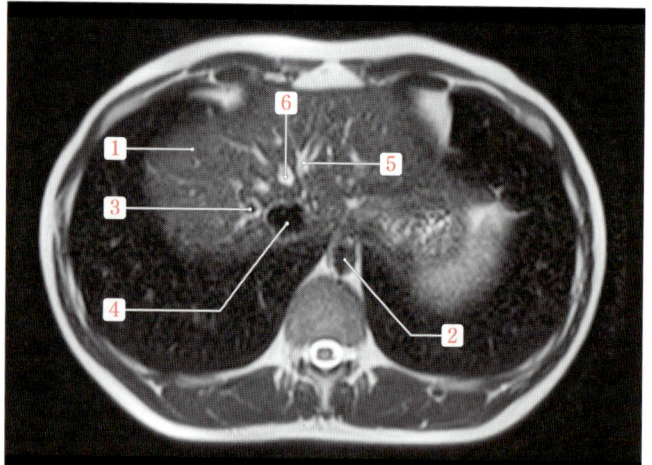

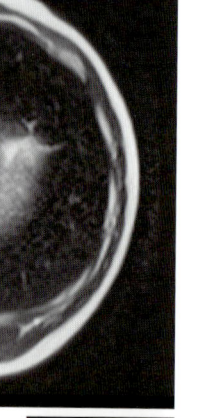

腹 部
Abdomen

MRI T2強調像（横断像）

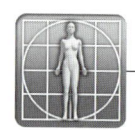

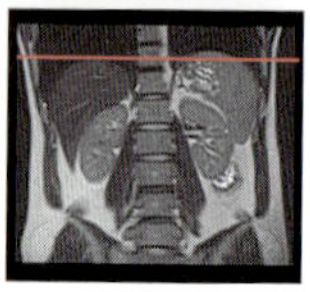

1 肝臓　Liver
2 下行大動脈　Descending aorta
3 右肝静脈　Right hepatic vein
4 下大静脈　Inferior vena cava
5 左肝静脈　Left hepatic vein
6 中肝静脈　Middle hepatic vein

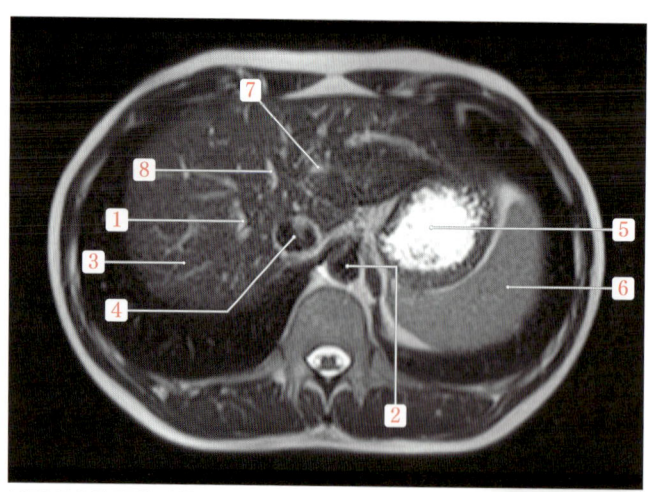

MRI T2強調像（横断像）

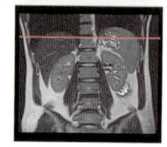

1 右肝静脈　Right hepatic vein
2 腹部大動脈　Abdominal aorta
3 肝臓　Liver
4 下大静脈　Inferior vena cava
5 胃　Stomach
6 脾臓　Spleen
7 左肝静脈　Left hepatic vein
8 中肝静脈　Middle hepatic vein

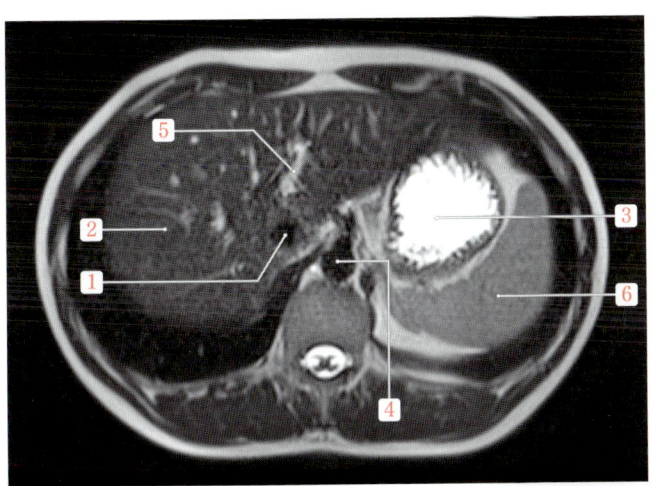

MRI T2強調像（横断像）

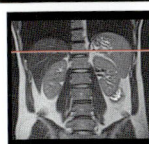

1 下大静脈　Inferior vena cava
2 肝臓　Liver
3 胃　Stomach
4 腹部大動脈　Abdominal aorta
5 門脈左枝　Left portal vein
6 脾臓　Spleen

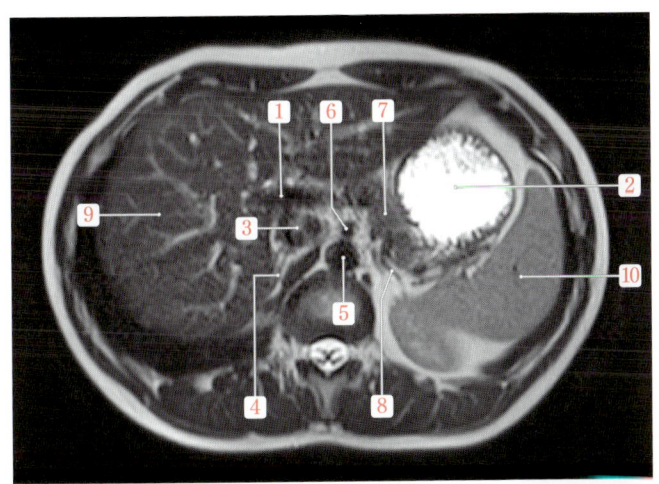

MRI T2強調像（横断像）

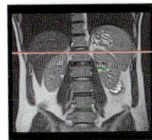

1 門脈本幹　Main portal vein
2 胃　Stomach
3 下大静脈　Inferior vena cava
4 右副腎　Right adrenal gland
5 腹部大動脈　Abdominal aorta
6 腹腔動脈　Celiac artery
7 膵臓　Pancreas
8 左副腎　Left adrenal gland
9 肝臓　Liver
10 脾臓　Spleen

腹部
Abdomen

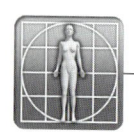

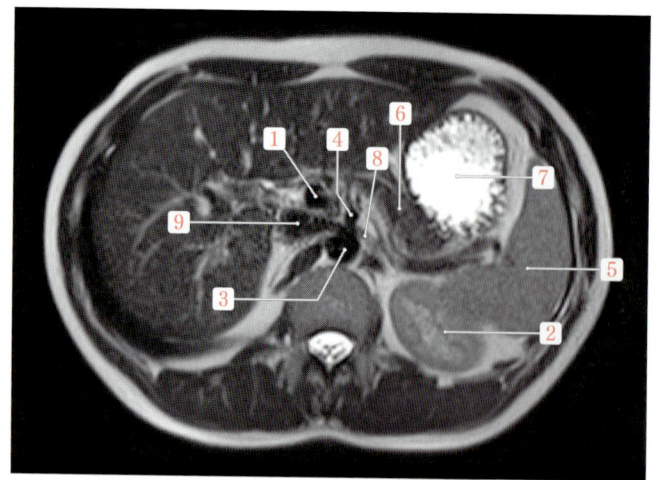

MRI T2強調像（横断像）

1 門脈本幹　Main portal vein
2 左腎　Left kidney
3 腹部大動脈　Abdominal aorta
4 上腸間膜動脈　Superior mesenteric artery
5 脾臓　Spleen
6 膵臓　Pancreas
7 胃　Stomach
8 左腎静脈　Left renal vein
9 下大静脈　Inferior vena cava

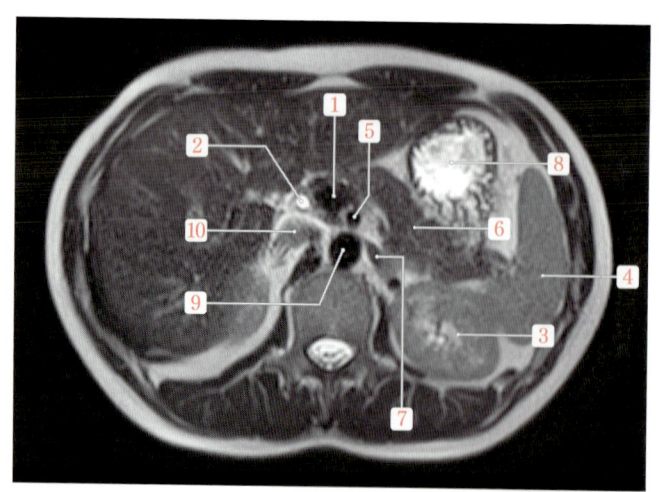

MRI T2強調像（横断像）

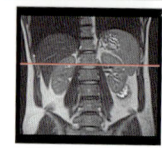

1 門脈本幹　Main portal vein
2 総胆管　Common bile duct
3 左腎　Left kidney
4 脾臓　Spleen
5 上腸間膜動脈　Superior mesenteric artery
6 膵臓　Pancreas
7 左腎静脈　Left renal vein
8 胃　Stomach
9 腹部大動脈　Abdominal aorta
10 下大静脈　Inferior vena cava

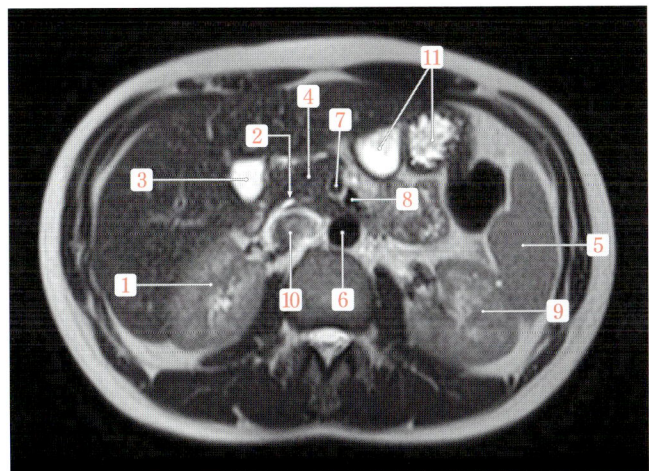

MRI T2強調像（横断像）

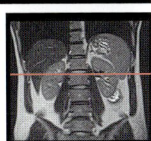

1　右腎　Right kidney
2　総胆管　Common bile duct
3　胆嚢　Gallbladder
4　膵臓　Pancreas
5　脾臓　Spleen
6　腹部大動脈　Abdominal aorta
7　上腸間膜静脈　Superior mesenteric vein
8　上腸間膜動脈
　　Superior mesenteric artery
9　左腎　Left kidney
10　下大静脈　Inferior vena cava
11　胃　Stomach

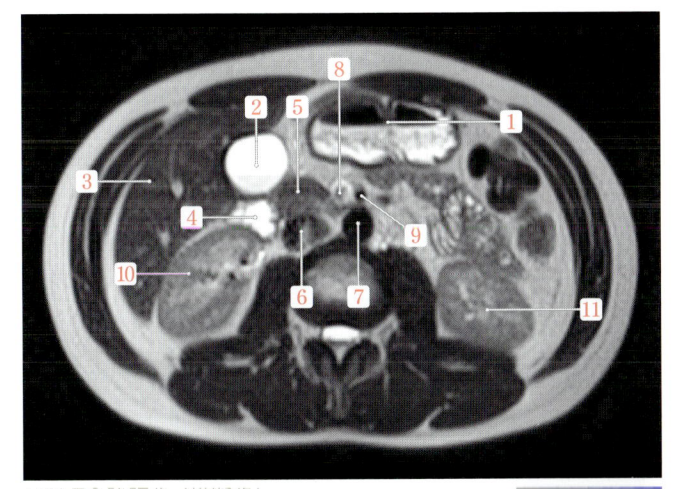

MRI T2強調像（横断像）

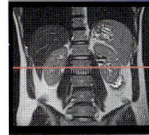

1　胃　Stomach
2　胆嚢　Gallbladder
3　肝臓　Liver
4　十二指腸　Duodenum
5　膵臓　Pancreas
6　下大静脈　Inferior vena cava
7　腹部大動脈　Abdominal aorta
8　上腸間膜静脈　Superior mesenteric vein
9　上腸間膜動脈
　　Superior mesenteric artery
10　右腎　Right kidney
11　左腎　Left kidney

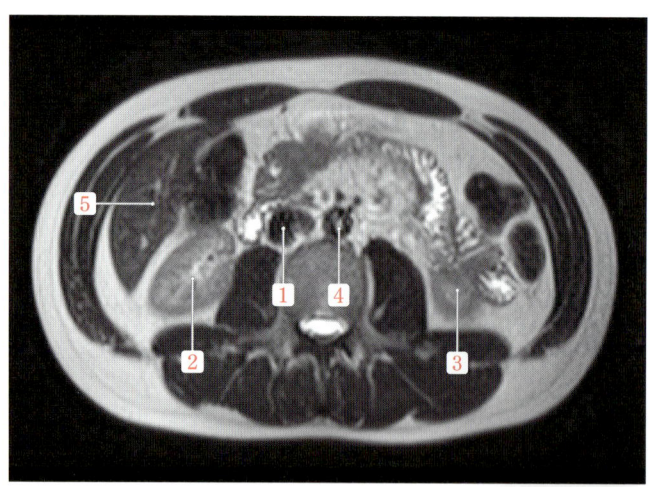

腹部
Abdomen

1 下大静脈　Inferior vena cava
2 右腎　Right kidney
3 左腎　Left kidney
4 腹部大動脈　Abdominal aorta
5 肝臓　Liver

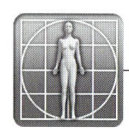

MRI T2強調像（横断像）

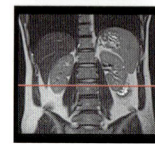

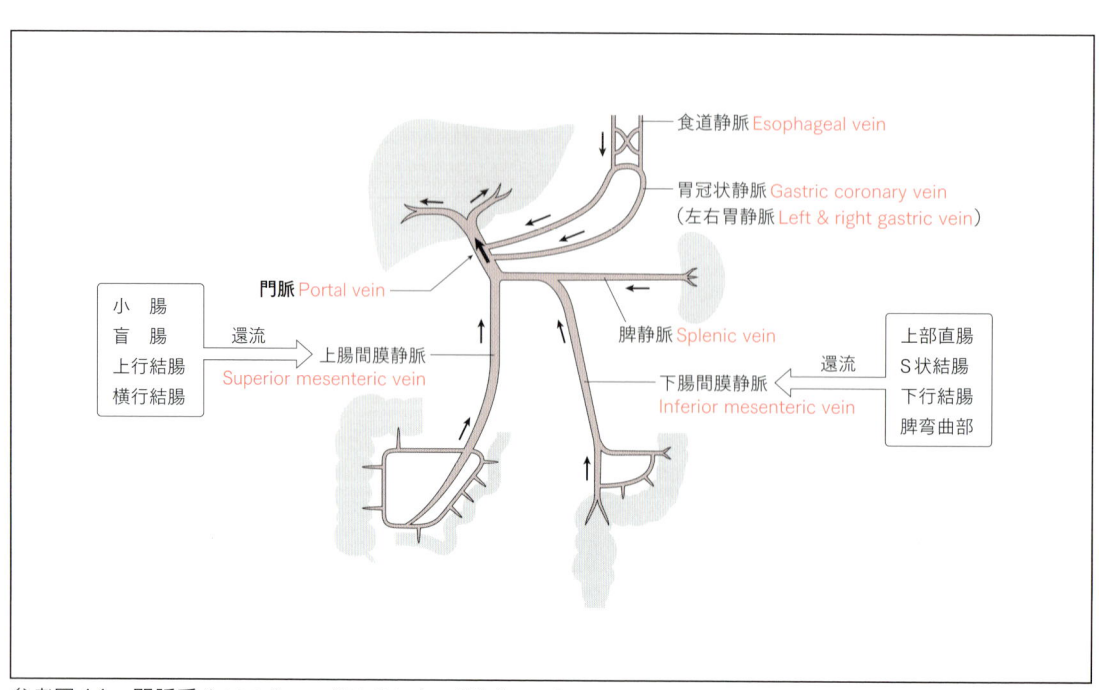

参考図11　門脈系（アイメディスン〈*i*Medicine〉7. 消化管. リブロ・サイエンス, 2010, p.30 より）

● CT・MRI 解体新書

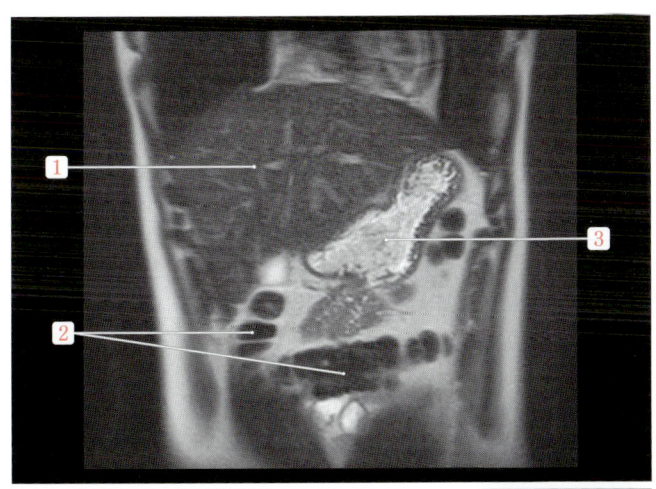

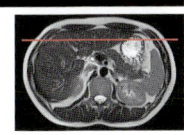

1 肝臓　Liver
2 結腸　Colon
3 胃　Stomach

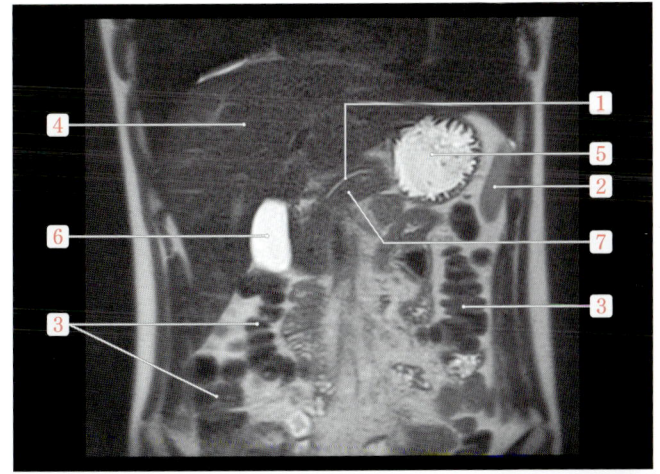

MRI T2 強調像（冠状断像）

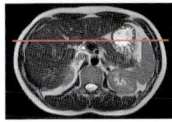

1 主膵管　Main pancreatic duct
2 脾臓　Spleen
3 結腸　Colon
4 肝臓　Liver
5 胃　Stomach
6 胆嚢　Gallbladder
7 膵臓　Pancreas

MRI T2 強調像（冠状断像）

腹部

89

腹部
Abdomen

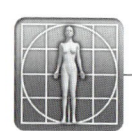

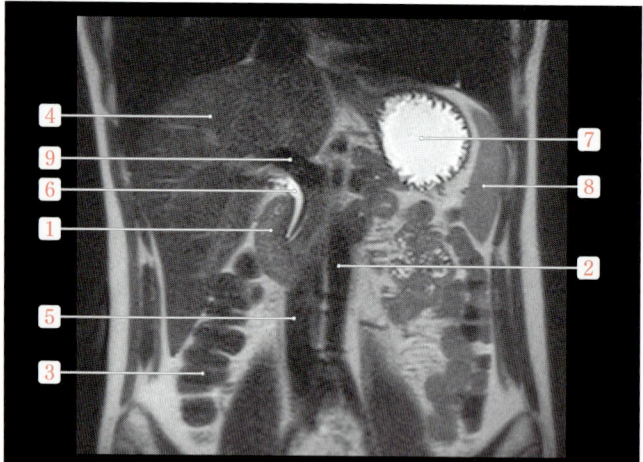

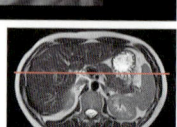

1 十二指腸　Duodenum
2 腹部大動脈　Abdominal aorta
3 上行結腸　Ascending colon
4 肝臓　Liver
5 下大静脈　Inferior vena cava
6 総胆管　Common bile duct
7 胃　Stomach
8 脾臓　Spleen
9 門脈　Portal vein

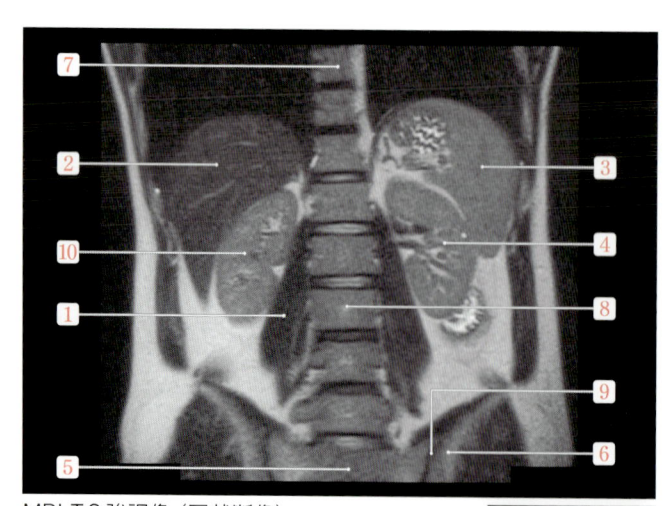

MRI T2強調像（冠状断像）

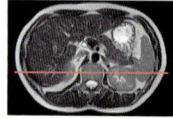

1 大腰筋　Psoas major
2 肝臓　Liver
3 脾臓　Spleen
4 左腎　Left kidney
5 仙椎　Sacral vertebra
6 腸骨　Ilium
7 胸椎　Thoracic vertebra
8 腰椎　Lumbar vertebra
9 仙腸関節　Sacro-iliac joint
10 右腎　Right kidney

MRI T2強調像（冠状断像）

●CT・MRI 解体新書

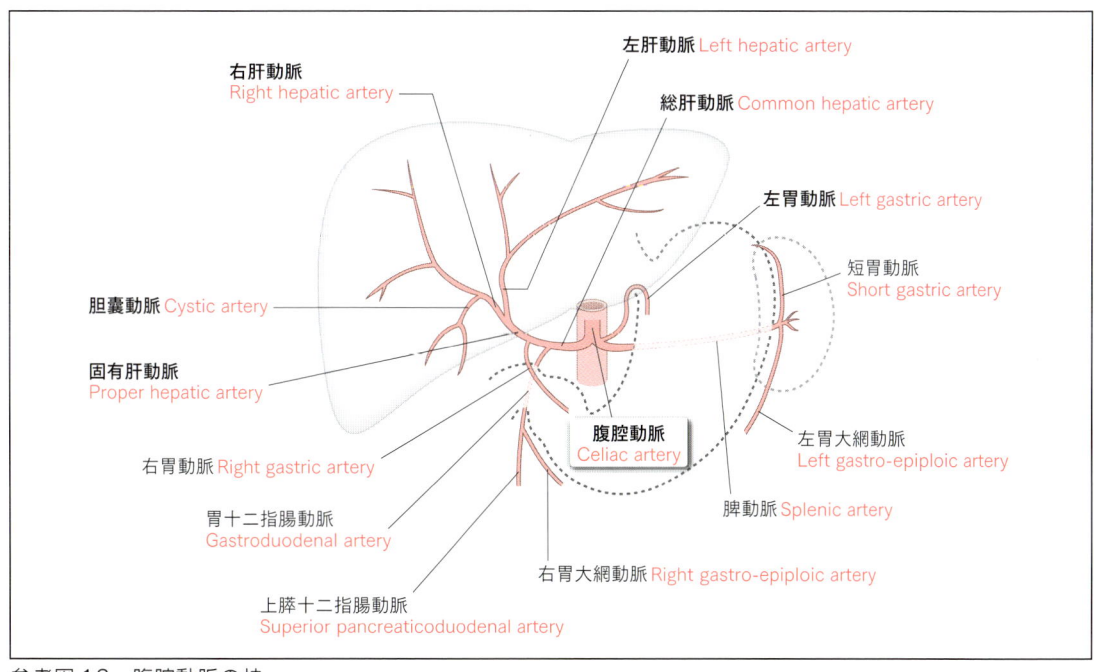

参考図12　腹腔動脈の枝

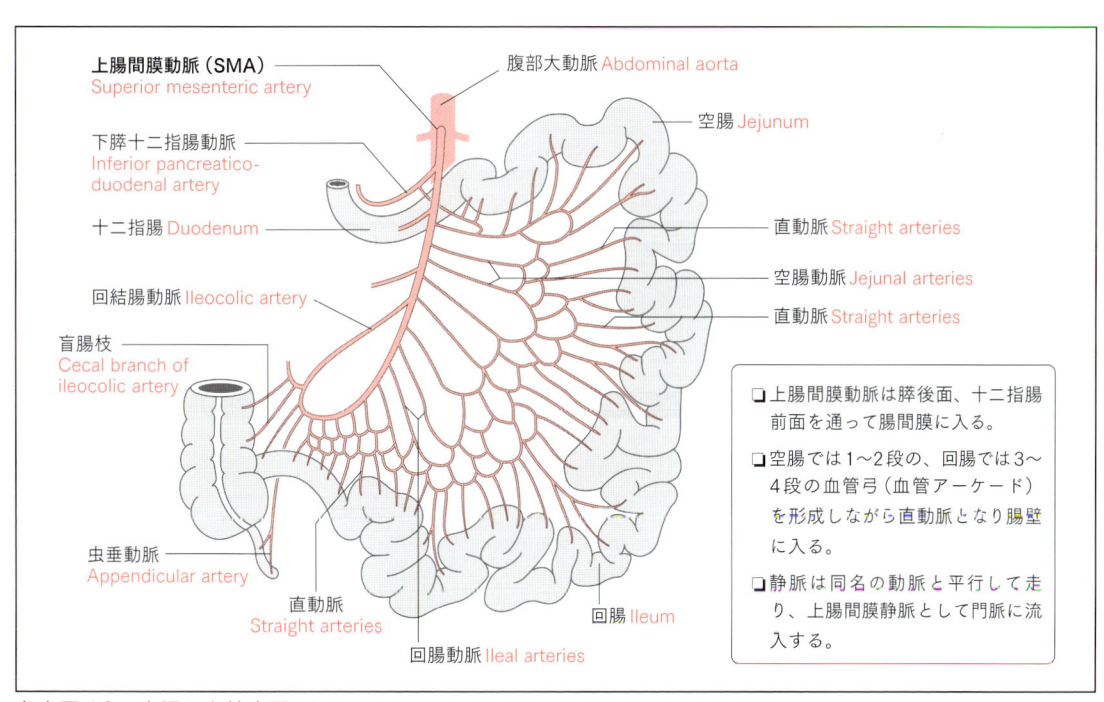

参考図13　小腸の血管支配（リブロ・サイエンス, *i*Medicine 7. 消化管, p.21 より引用）

- 上腸間膜動脈は膵後面、十二指腸前面を通って腸間膜に入る。
- 空腸では1〜2段の、回腸では3〜4段の血管弓（血管アーケード）を形成しながら直動脈となり腸壁に入る。
- 静脈は同名の動脈と平行して走り、上腸間膜静脈として門脈に流入する。

腹部

91

腹 部
Abdomen

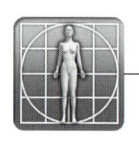

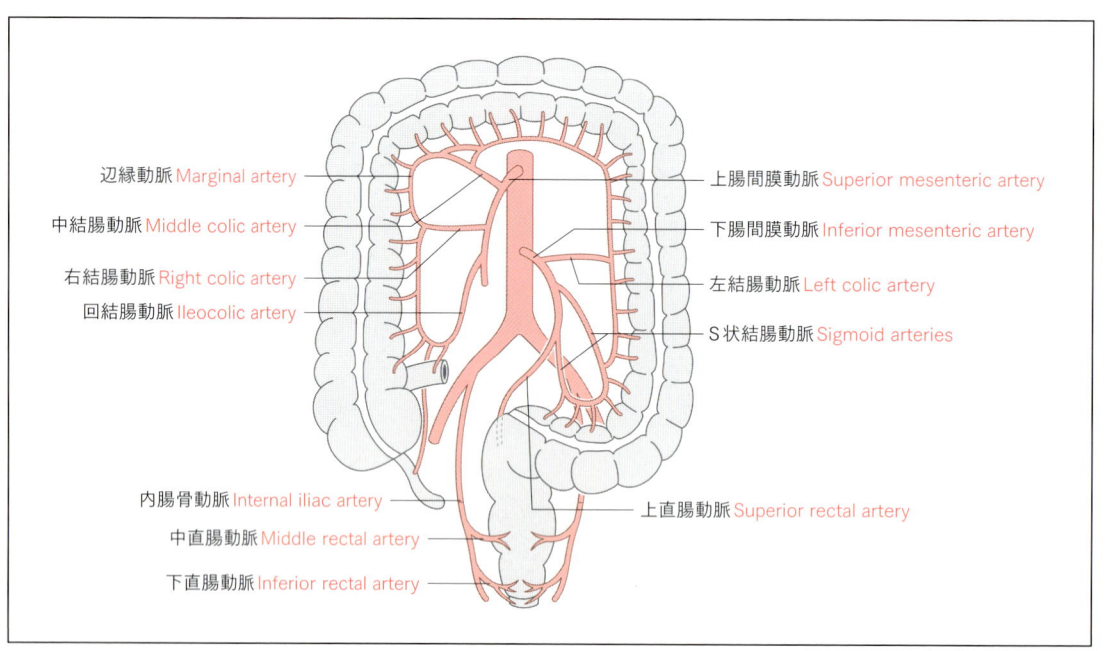

参考図14　大腸の血管支配（アイメディスン〈*i*Medicine〉7. 消化管. リブロ・サイエンス, 2010, p.22 より）

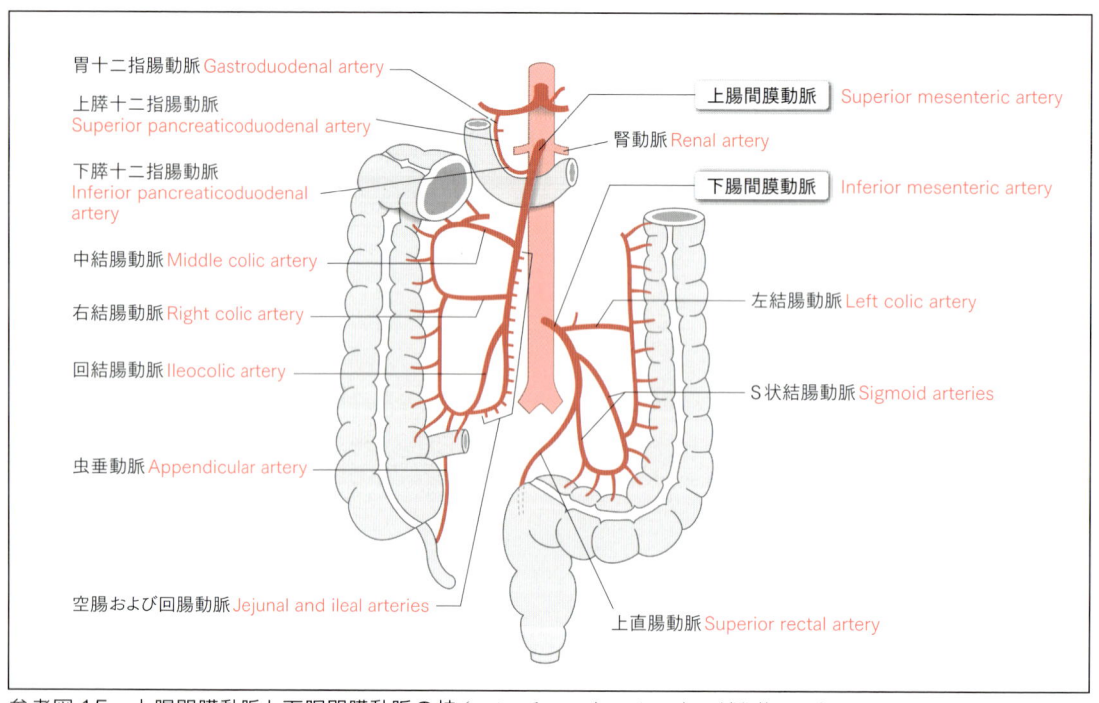

- 辺縁動脈 Marginal artery
- 中結腸動脈 Middle colic artery
- 右結腸動脈 Right colic artery
- 回結腸動脈 Ileocolic artery
- 内腸骨動脈 Internal iliac artery
- 中直腸動脈 Middle rectal artery
- 下直腸動脈 Inferior rectal artery
- 上腸間膜動脈 Superior mesenteric artery
- 下腸間膜動脈 Inferior mesenteric artery
- 左結腸動脈 Left colic artery
- S状結腸動脈 Sigmoid arteries
- 上直腸動脈 Superior rectal artery

参考図15　上腸間膜動脈と下腸間膜動脈の枝（アイメディスン〈*i*Medicine〉7. 消化管. リブロ・サイエンス, 2010, p.29 より）

- 胃十二指腸動脈 Gastroduodenal artery
- 上膵十二指腸動脈 Superior pancreaticoduodenal artery
- 下膵十二指腸動脈 Inferior pancreaticoduodenal artery
- 中結腸動脈 Middle colic artery
- 右結腸動脈 Right colic artery
- 回結腸動脈 Ileocolic artery
- 虫垂動脈 Appendicular artery
- 空腸および回腸動脈 Jejunal and ileal arteries
- 上腸間膜動脈 Superior mesenteric artery
- 腎動脈 Renal artery
- 下腸間膜動脈 Inferior mesenteric artery
- 左結腸動脈 Left colic artery
- S状結腸動脈 Sigmoid arteries
- 上直腸動脈 Superior rectal artery

CT・MRI
解体新書
- 正常解剖 -

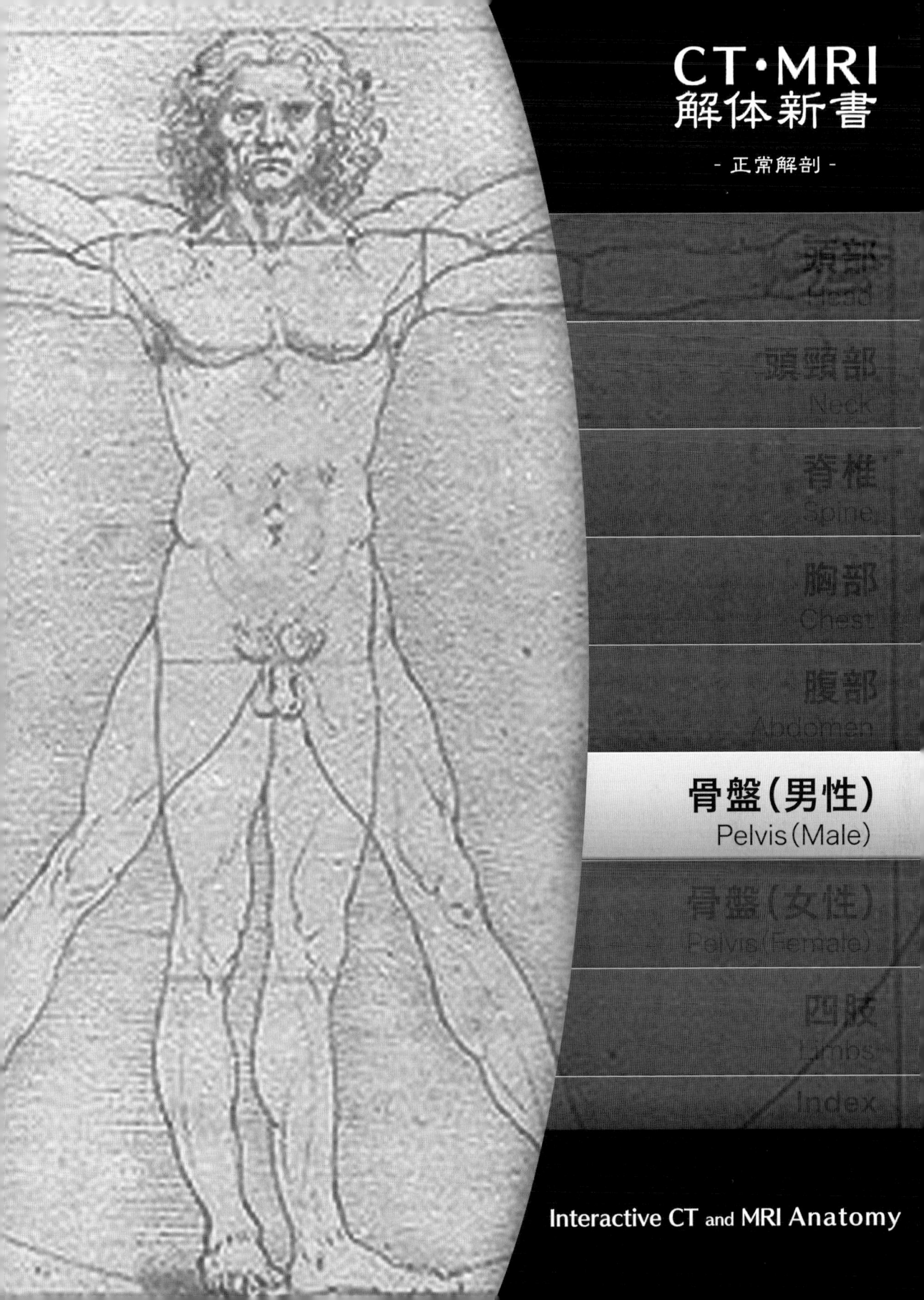

頭部 Head

頭頸部 Neck

脊椎 Spine

胸部 Chest

腹部 Abdomen

骨盤（男性）
Pelvis (Male)

骨盤（女性） Pelvis (Female)

四肢 Limbs

Index

Interactive CT and MRI Anatomy

骨盤（男性）
Pelvis (Male)

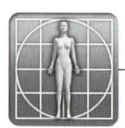

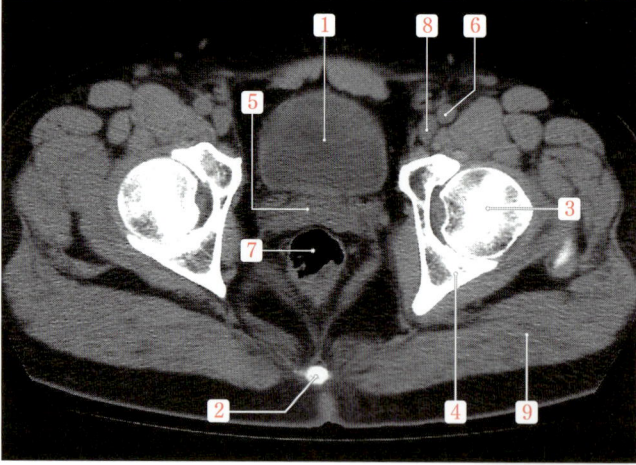

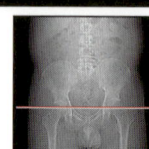

1 膀胱　Urinary bladder
2 尾骨　Coccyx
3 大腿骨頭　Femoral head
4 坐骨　Ischium
5 精嚢　Seminal vesicle
6 大腿動脈　Femoral artery
7 直腸　Rectum
8 大腿静脈　Femoral vein
9 大殿筋　Gluteus maximus

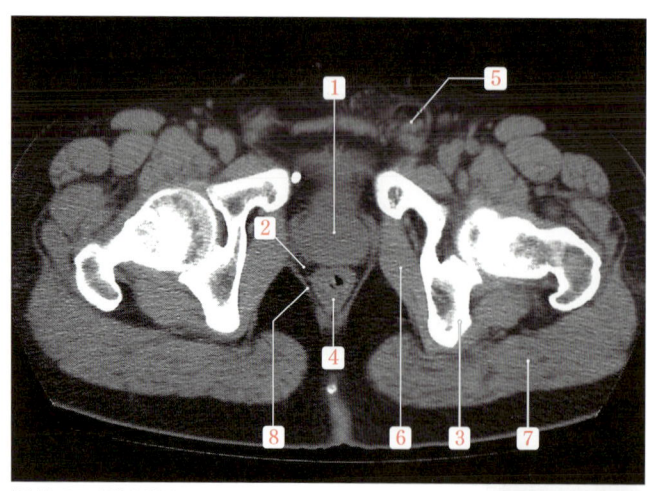

単純CT（横断像）

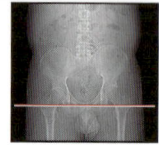

1 前立腺　Prostate
2 直腸周囲腔　Perirectal space
3 坐骨　Ischium
4 直腸　Rectum
5 精索　Spermatic cord
6 内閉鎖筋　Internal obturator
7 大殿筋　Gluteus maximus
8 肛門挙筋　Levator ani

単純CT（横断像）

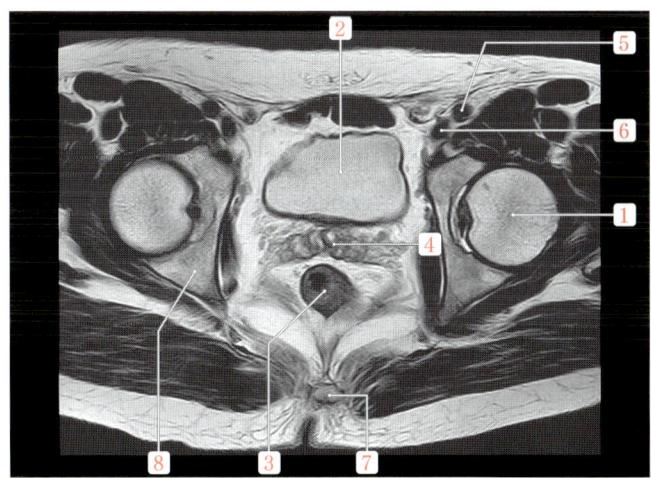

● CT・MRI 解体新書

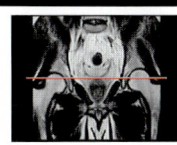

1 大腿骨頭　Femoral head
2 膀胱　Urinary bladder
3 直腸　Rectum
4 精囊　Seminal vesicle
5 大腿動脈　Femoral artery
6 大腿静脈　Femoral vein
7 尾骨　Coccyx
8 坐骨　Ischium

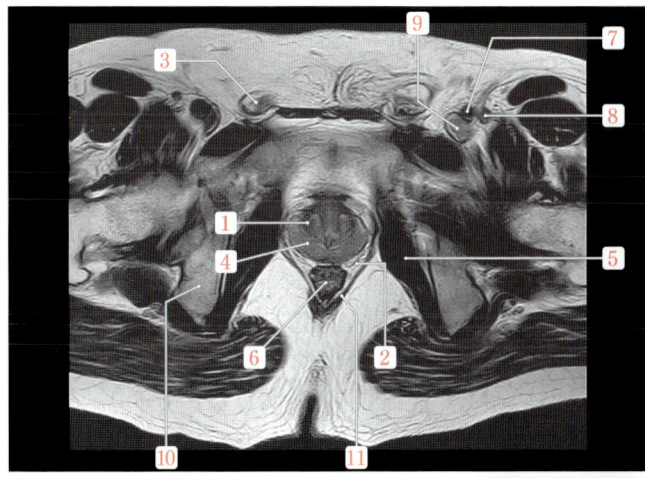

MRI T2 強調像（横断像）

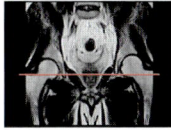

1 前立腺（中心域）　Prostate (central zone)
2 直腸周囲腔　Perirectal space
3 精索　Spermatic cord
4 前立腺（辺縁域）
　 Prostate (peripheral zone)
5 内閉鎖筋　Internal obturator
6 直腸　Rectum
7 浅大腿動脈　Superficial femoral artery
8 深大腿動脈　Deep femoral artery
9 大腿静脈　Femoral vein
10 坐骨　Ischium
11 肛門挙筋　Levator ani

MRI T2 強調像（横断像）

骨盤（男性）

95

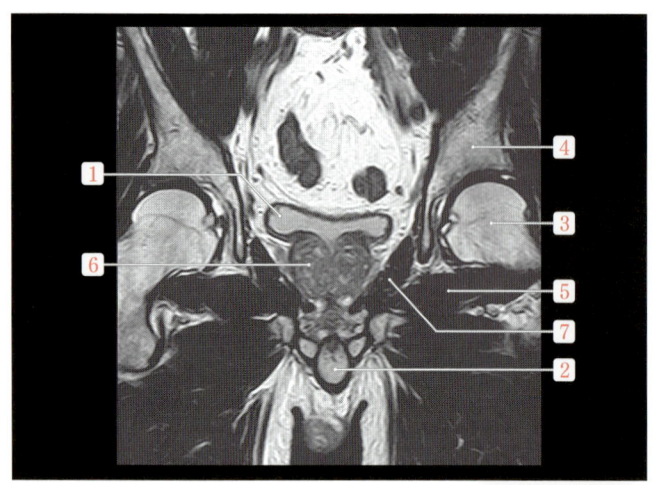

骨盤（男性）
Pelvis (Male)

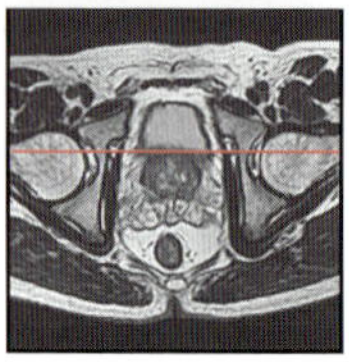

1 膀胱　Urinary bladder
2 陰茎　Penis
3 大腿骨頭　Femoral head
4 寛骨臼蓋　Acetabular roof
5 外閉鎖筋　External obturator
6 前立腺　Prostate
7 内閉鎖筋　Internal obturator

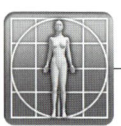

MRI T2強調像（冠状断像）

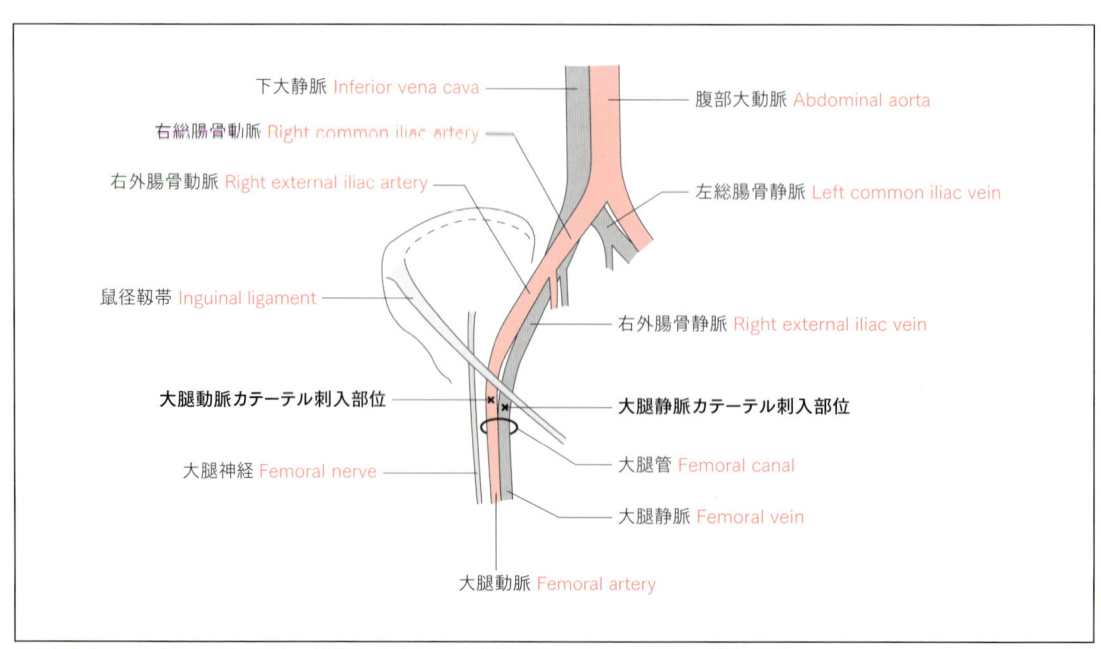

参考図16　大腿部の動静脈・神経の走行と大腿動静脈へのカテーテル刺入部位
（アイメディスン〈*i*Medicine〉1. 循環器．リブロ・サイエンス，2008，p.26より）

CT・MRI 解体新書

- 正常解剖 -

頭部 Head

頭頸部 Neck

脊椎 Spine

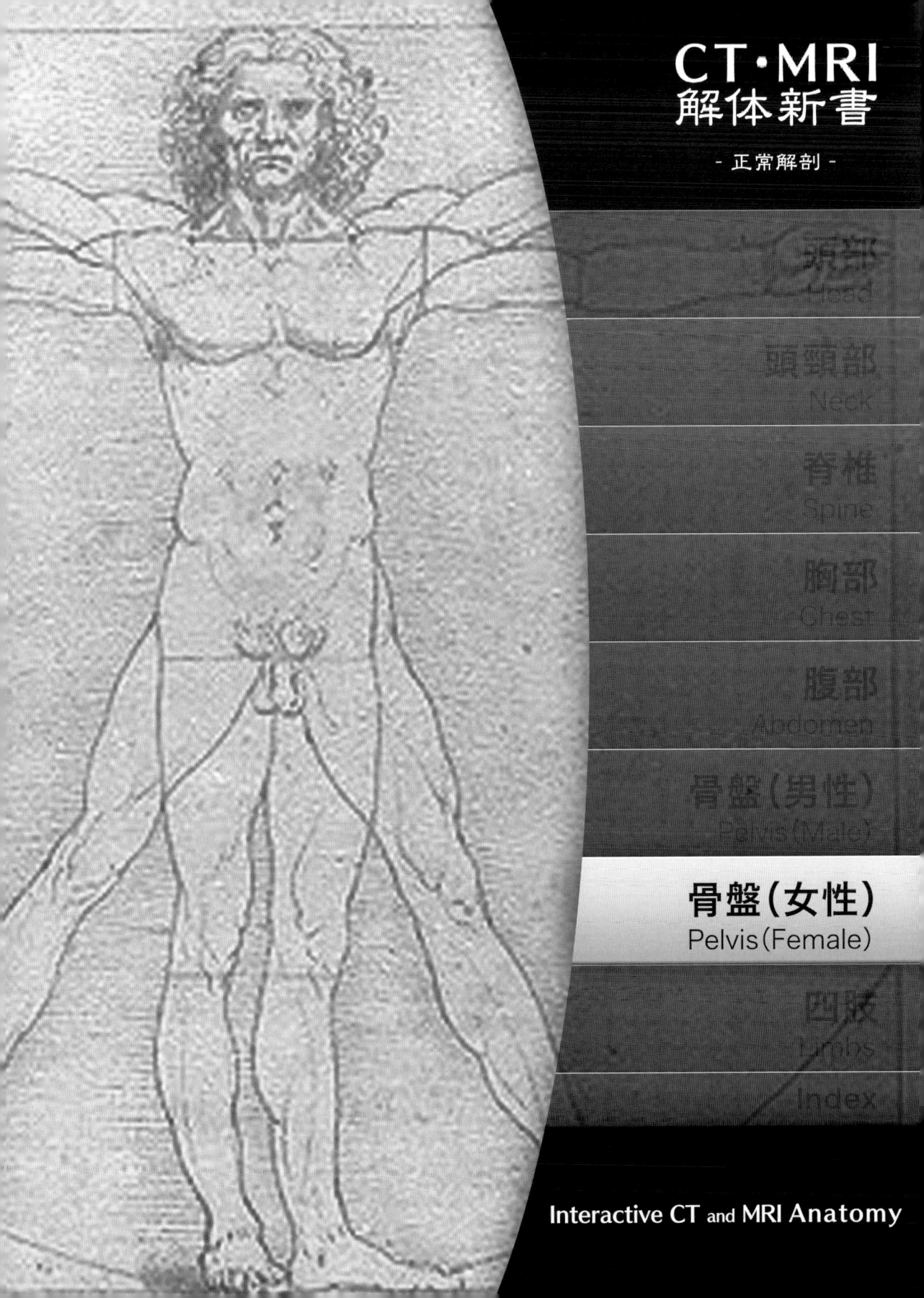

胸部 Chest

腹部 Abdomen

骨盤(男性) Pelvis(Male)

骨盤(女性) Pelvis(Female)

四肢 Limbs

Index

Interactive CT and MRI Anatomy

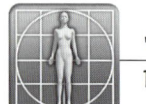

骨盤（女性）
Pelvis (Female)

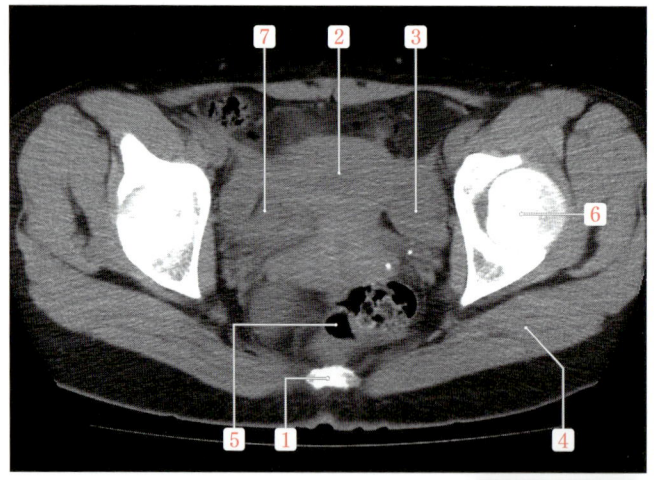

1 尾骨　Coccyx
2 子宮　Uterus
3 左卵巣　Left ovary
4 大殿筋　Gluteus maximus
5 直腸　Rectum
6 大腿骨頭　Femoral head
7 右卵巣　Right ovary

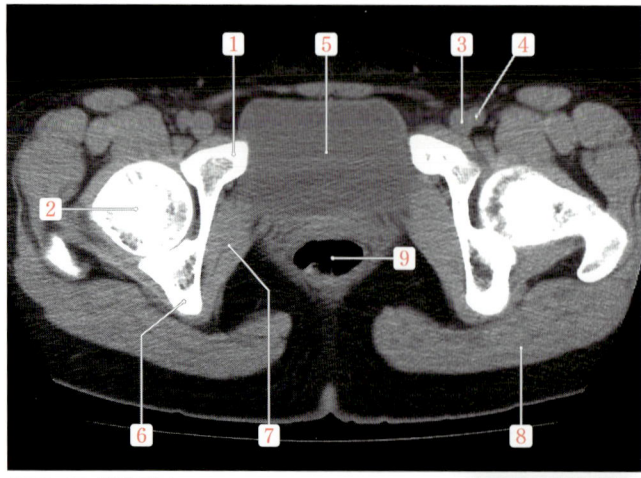

単純CT（横断像）

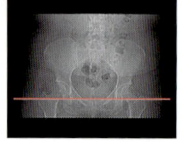

1 恥骨　Pubis
2 大腿骨頭　Femoral head
3 大腿静脈　Femoral vein
4 大腿動脈　Femoral artery
5 膀胱　Urinary bladder
6 坐骨　Ischium
7 内閉鎖筋　Internal obturator
8 大殿筋　Gluteus maximus
9 直腸　Rectum

単純CT（横断像）

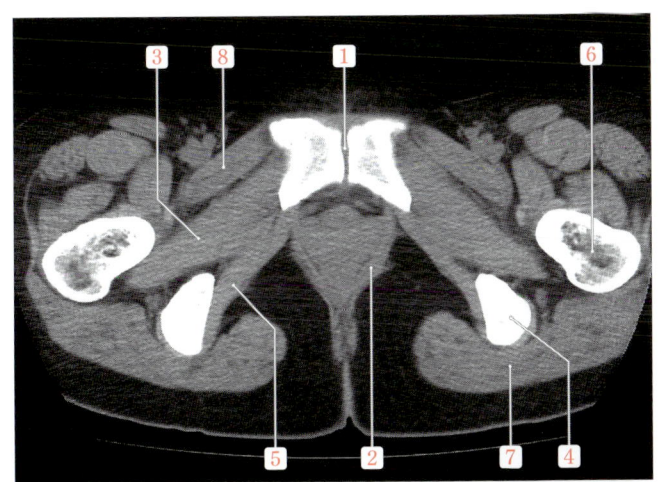

単純CT（横断像）

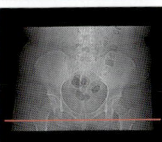

1 恥骨結合　Pubic symphysis
2 肛門挙筋　Levator ani
3 外閉鎖筋　External obturator
4 坐骨　Ischium
5 内閉鎖筋　Internal obturator
6 大腿骨　Femur
7 大殿筋　Gluteus maximus
8 恥骨筋　Pectineus

骨盤（女性）
Pelvis (Female)

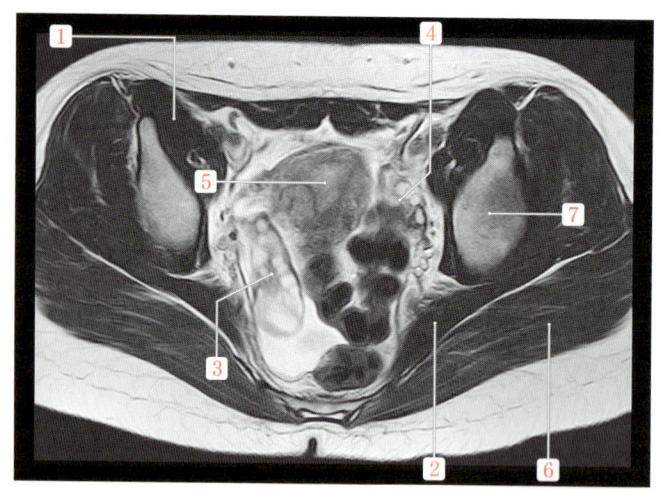

1 腸腰筋　Iliopsoas
2 梨状筋　Piriformis
3 右卵巣　Right ovary
4 左卵巣　Left ovary
5 子宮体部　Uterine body
6 大殿筋　Gluteus maximus
7 腸骨　Ilium

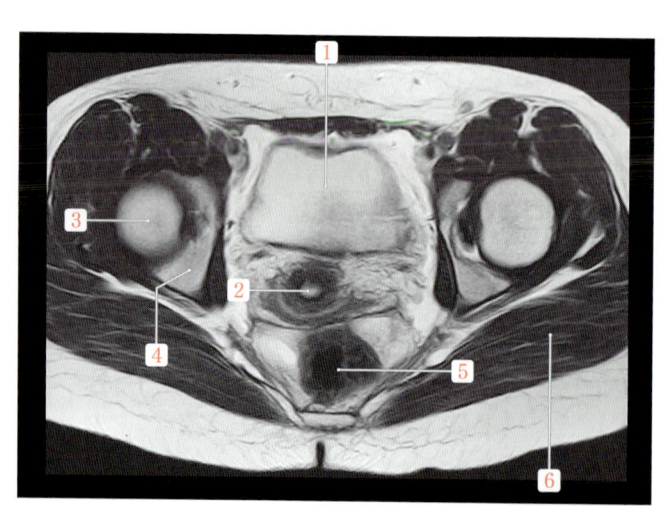

MRI T2強調像（横断像）

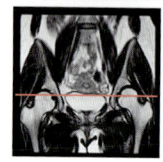

1 膀胱　Urinary bladder
2 子宮頸部　Uterine cervix
3 大腿骨頭　Femoral head
4 坐骨　Ischium
5 直腸　Rectum
6 大殿筋　Gluteus maximus

MRI T2強調像（横断像）

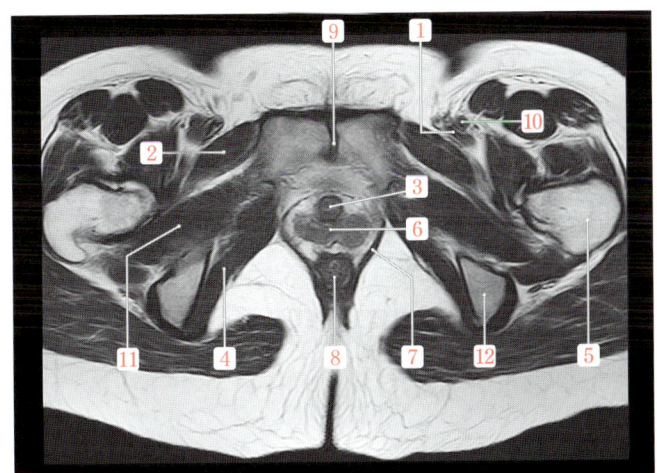

MRI T2強調像（横断像）

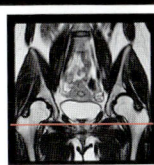

1　大腿静脈　Femoral vein
2　恥骨筋　Pectineus
3　尿道　Urethra
4　内閉鎖筋　Internal obturator
5　大腿骨　Femur
6　膣　Vagina
7　肛門挙筋　Levator ani
8　肛門　Anus
9　恥骨結合　Pubic symphysis
10　大腿動脈　Femoral artery
11　外閉鎖筋　External obturator
12　坐骨　Ischium

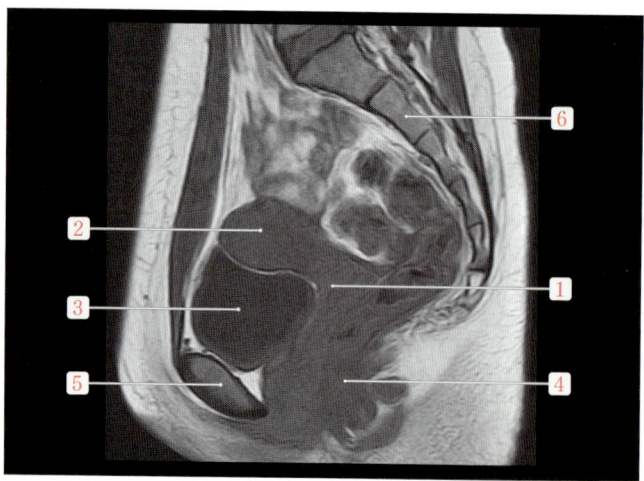

骨盤（女性）
Pelvis (Female)

1 子宮頸部　Uterine cervix
2 子宮体部　Uterine body
3 膀胱　Urinary bladder
4 直腸　Rectum
5 恥骨　Pubis
6 仙骨　Sacrum

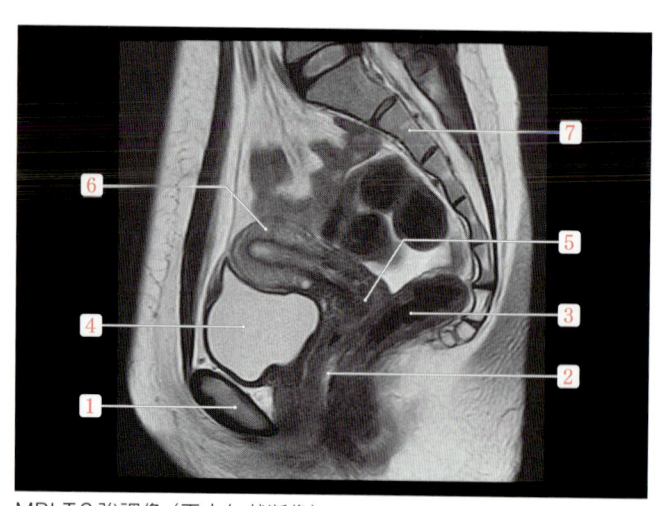

MRI T1 強調像（正中矢状断像）

1 恥骨　Pubis
2 腟　Vagina
3 直腸　Rectum
4 膀胱　Urinary bladder
5 子宮頸部　Uterine cervix
6 子宮体部　Uterine body
7 仙骨　Sacrum

MRI T2 強調像（正中矢状断像）

CT・MRI 解体新書
- 正常解剖 -

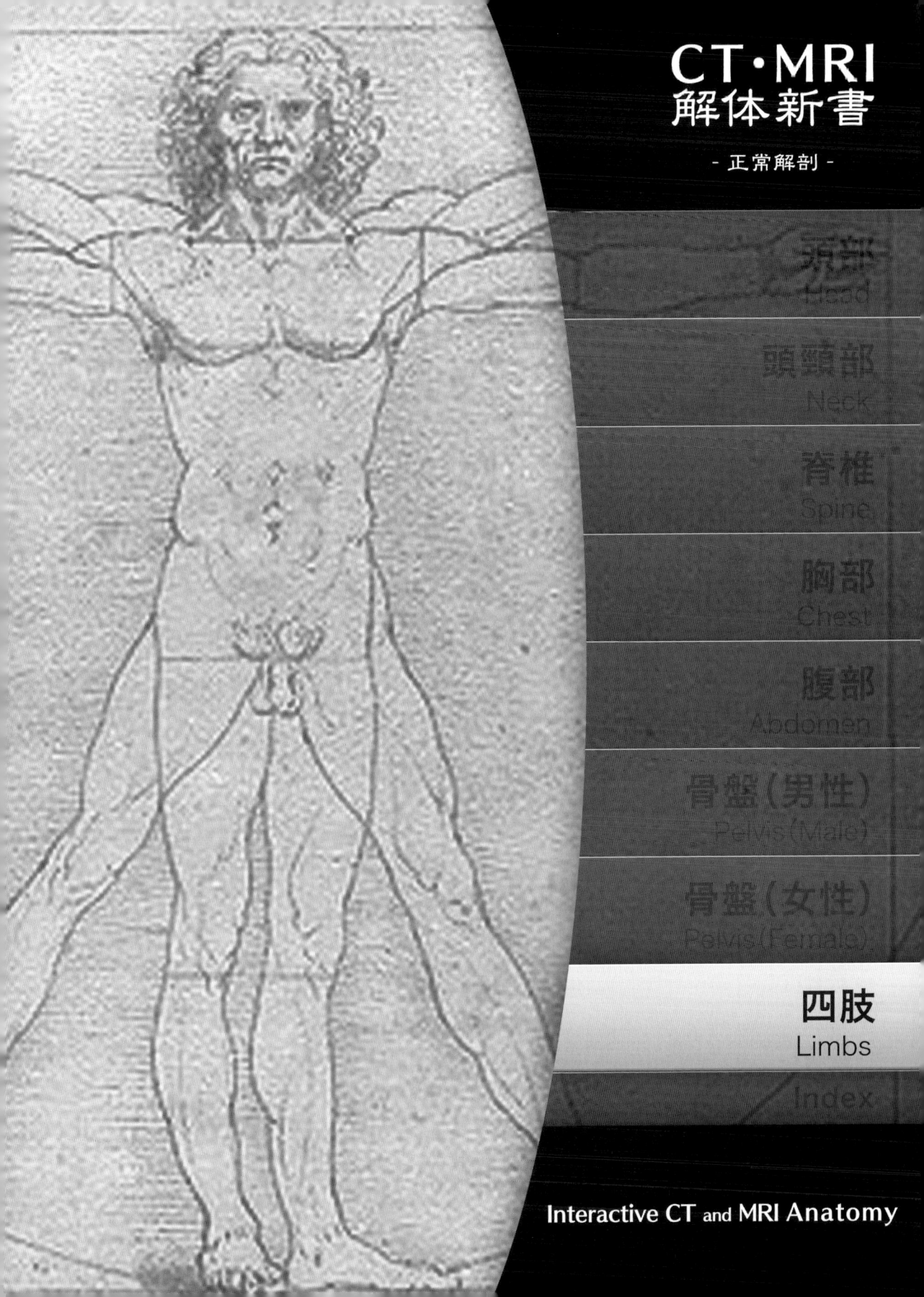

頭部 Head

頭頸部 Neck

脊椎 Spine

胸部 Chest

腹部 Abdomen

骨盤(男性) Pelvis (Male)

骨盤(女性) Pelvis (Female)

四肢 Limbs

Index

Interactive CT and MRI Anatomy

四 肢
Limbs

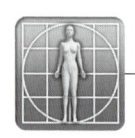

肩 Shoulder

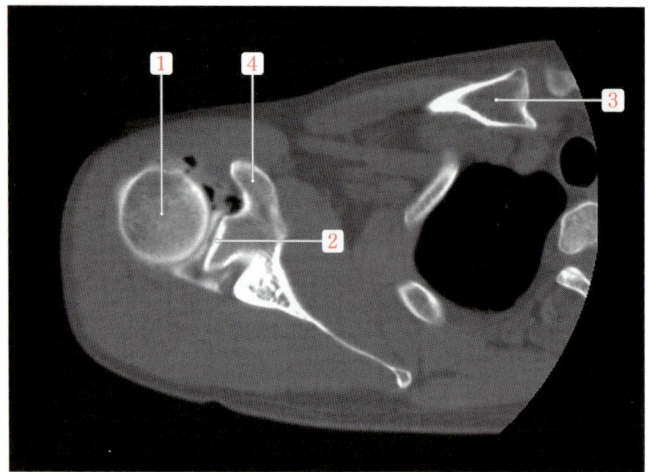

アルトロCT（横断像）

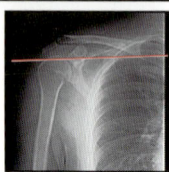

1 上腕骨頭　Humeral head
2 肩甲骨関節窩　Glenoid cavity of scapula
3 鎖骨　Clavicle
4 烏口突起　Coracoid process

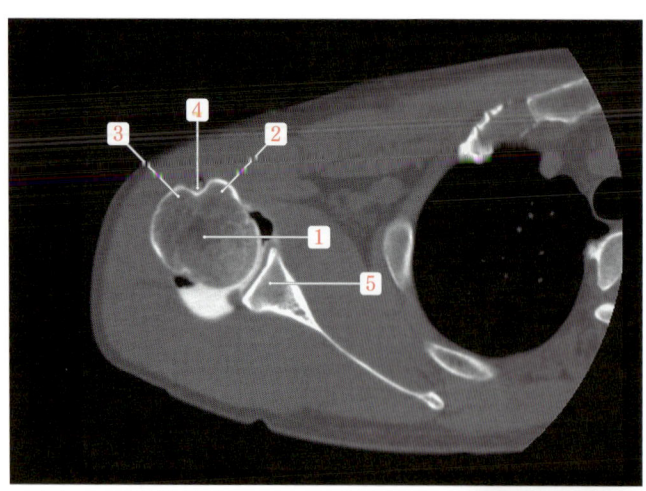

アルトロCT（横断像）

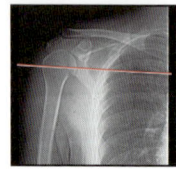

1 上腕骨頭　Humeral head
2 小結節　Lesser tubercle
3 大結節　Greater tubercle
4 結節間溝　Intertubercular sulcus
5 肩甲骨関節窩　Glenoid cavity of scapula

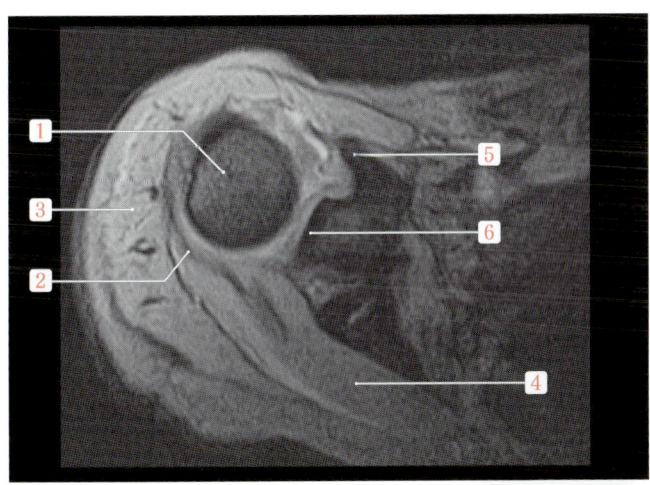

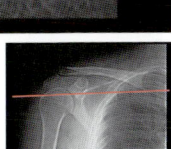

1　上腕骨頭　Humeral head
2　棘下筋腱　Infraspinatus tendon
3　三角筋　Deltoid
4　棘下筋　Infraspinatus
5　烏口突起　Coracoid process
6　肩甲骨関節窩　Glenoid cavity of scapula

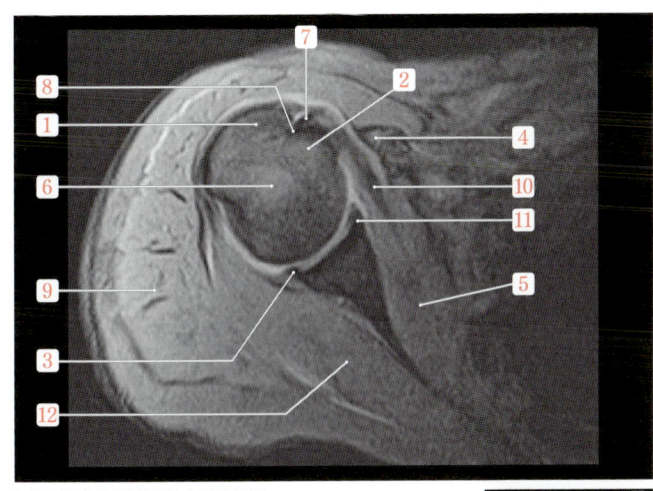

MRI T2*強調像（横断像）

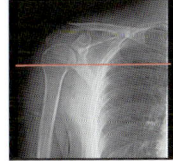

1　大結節　Greater tubercle
2　小結節　Lesser tubercle
3　後関節唇　Posterior labrum
4　烏口突起　Coracoid process
5　肩甲下筋　Subscapularis
6　上腕骨頭　Humeral head
7　上腕二頭筋長頭腱　Long head of biceps brachii tendon
8　結節間溝　Intertubercular sulcus
9　三角筋　Deltoid
10　肩甲下筋腱　Subscapularis tendon
11　前関節唇　Anterior labrum
12　棘下筋　Infraspinatus

MRI T2*強調像（横断像）

● CT・MRI 解体新書

四肢

105

四 肢
Limbs

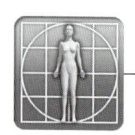

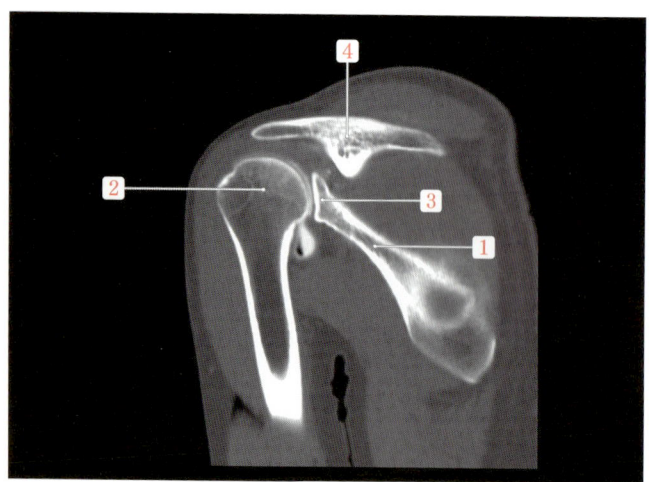

アルトロCT（斜位冠状断像）

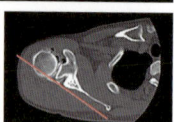

1 肩甲棘　Scapular spine
2 上腕骨頭　Humeral head
3 肩甲骨関節窩　Glenoid cavity of scapula
4 肩峰　Acromion

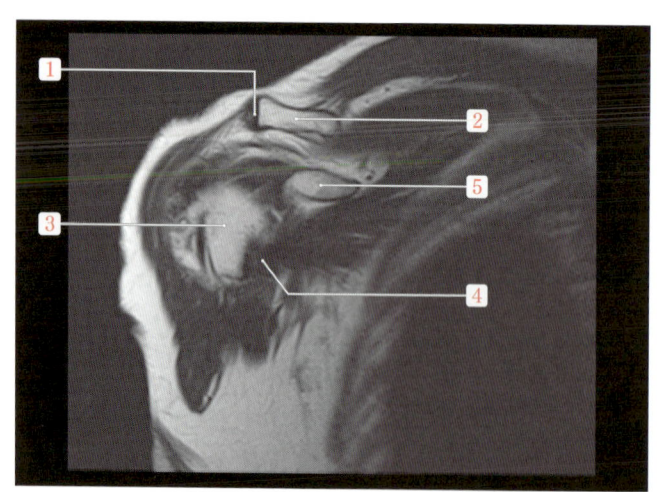

MRI T2強調像（斜位冠状断像）

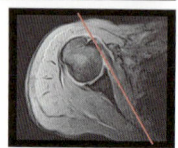

1 肩鎖関節　Acromioclavicular joint
2 鎖骨　Clavicle
3 上腕骨頭　Humeral head
4 肩甲下筋　Subscapularis
5 烏口突起　Coracoid process

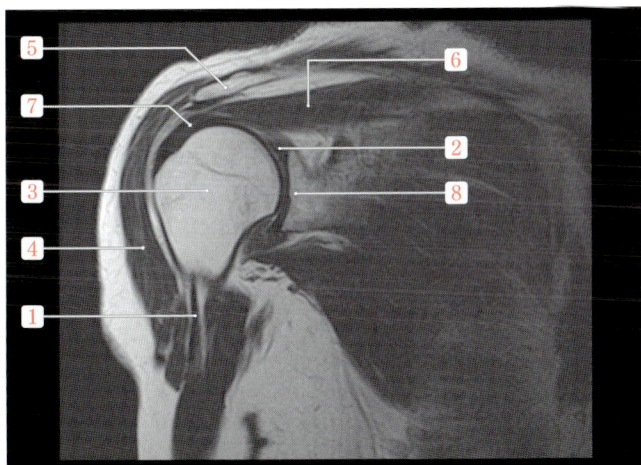

● CT・MRI 解体新書

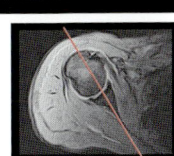

1 上腕二頭筋長頭腱
　Long head of biceps brachii tendon
2 関節唇　Labrum
3 上腕骨頭　Humeral head
4 三角筋　Deltoid
5 肩峰　Acromion
6 棘上筋　Supraspinatus
7 棘上筋腱　Supraspinatus tendon
8 肩甲骨関節窩　Glenoid cavity of scapula

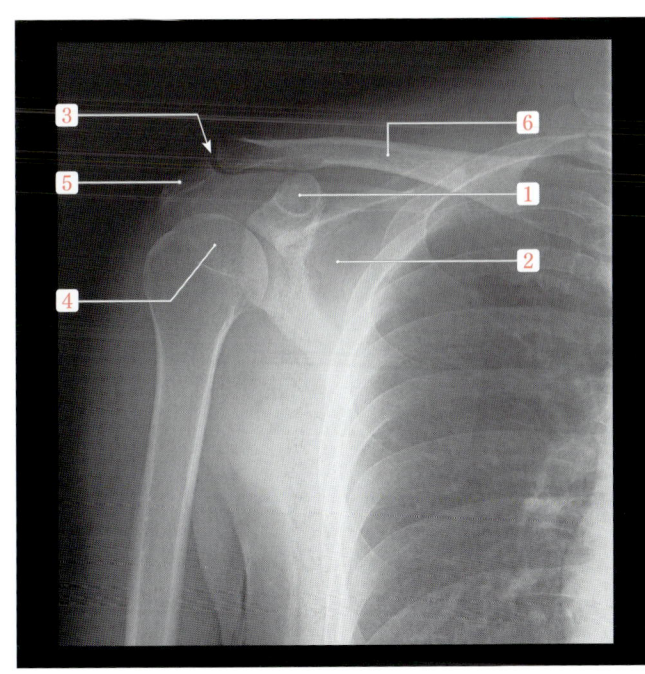

MRI T2強調像（斜位冠状断像）

1 烏口突起　Coracoid process
2 肩甲骨　Scapula
3 肩鎖関節　Acromioclavicular joint
4 上腕骨頭　Humeral head
5 肩峰　Acromion
6 鎖骨　Clavicle

単純X線

四肢

107

四 肢
Limbs

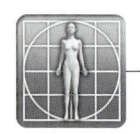

肘 Elbow

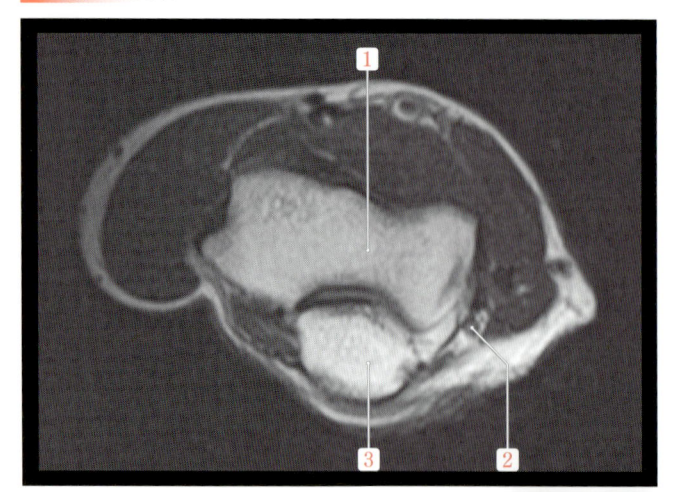

1 上腕骨　Humerus
2 尺骨神経　Ulnar nerve
3 肘頭　Olecranon

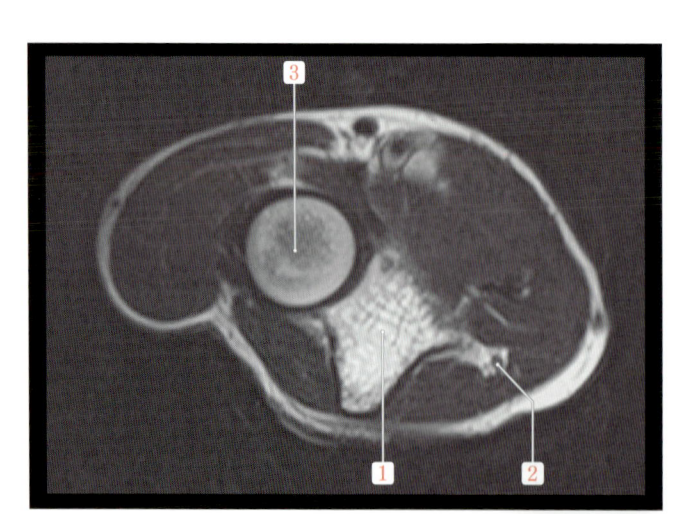

MRI T2強調像（横断像）

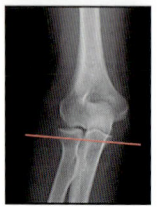

1 尺骨　Ulna
2 尺骨神経　Ulnar nerve
3 橈骨頭　Head of radius

MRI T2強調像（横断像）

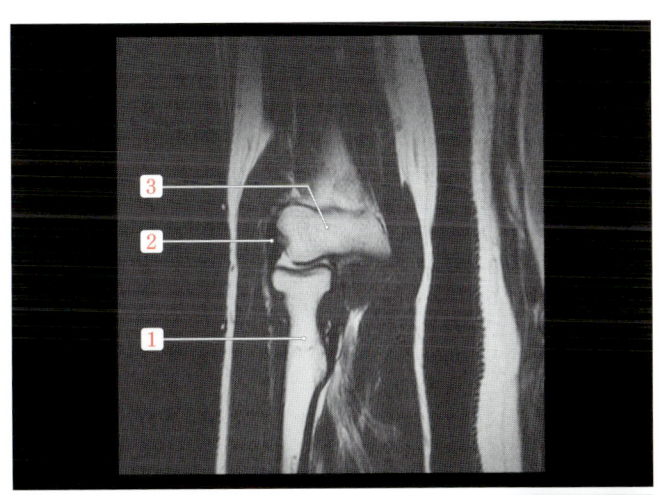

1　橈骨　Radius
2　外側側副靱帯　Lateral collateral ligament
3　上腕骨　Humerus

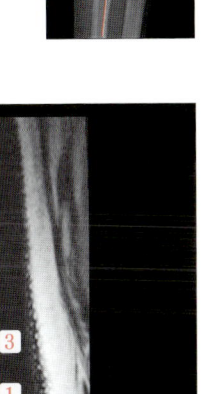

MRI T2強調像（冠状断像）

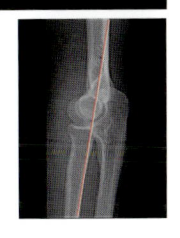

1　尺骨　Ulna
2　上腕骨　Humerus
3　内側側副靱帯　Medial collateral ligament
4　橈骨　Radius

MRI T2強調像（冠状断像）

四 肢
Limbs

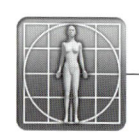

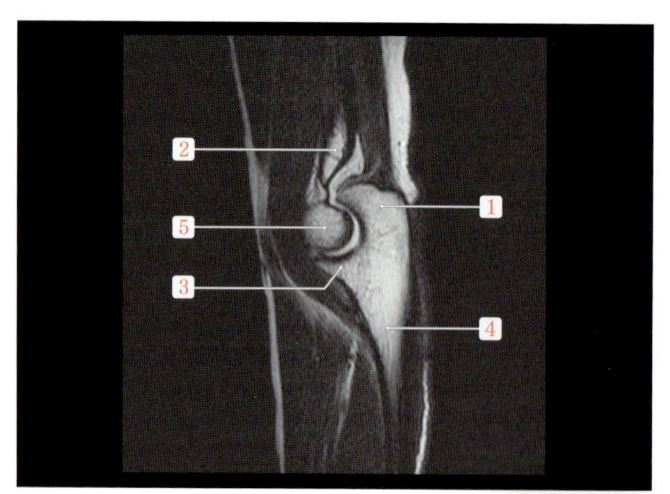

1　肘頭　Olecranon
2　上腕骨　Humerus
3　鈎状突起　Coronoid process
4　尺骨　Ulna
5　上腕骨滑車　Trochlea

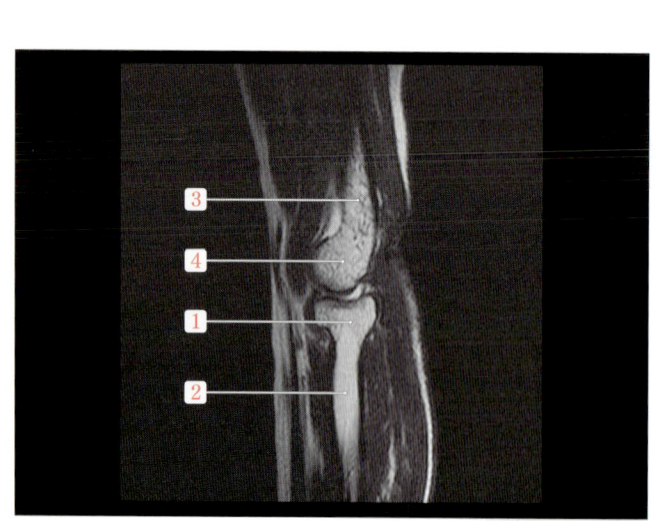

MRI T2強調像（矢状断像）

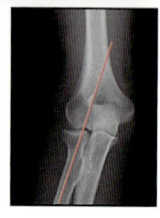

1　橈骨頭　Head of radius
2　橈骨　Radius
3　上腕骨　Humerus
4　上腕骨小頭　Capitulum

MRI T2強調像（矢状断像）

110

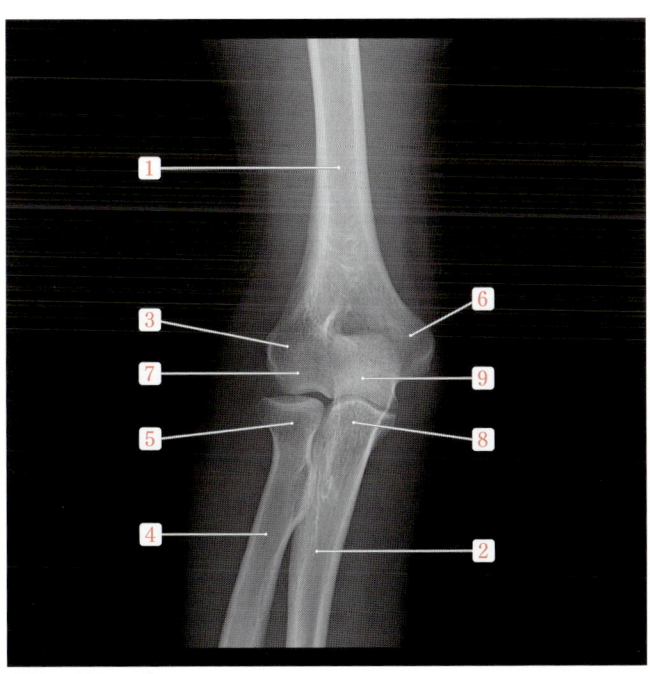

1 上腕骨　Humerus
2 尺骨　Ulna
3 外側上顆　Lateral epicondyle
4 橈骨　Radius
5 橈骨頭　Head of radius
6 内側上顆　Medial epicondyle
7 上腕骨小頭　Capitulum
8 鉤状突起　Coronoid process
9 上腕骨滑車　Trochlea

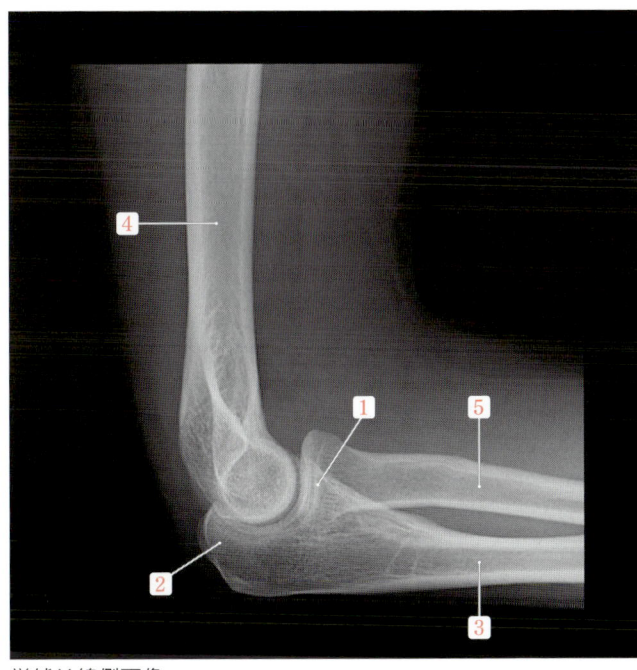

単純X線正面像

1 橈骨頭　Head of radius
2 肘頭　Olecranon
3 尺骨　Ulna
4 上腕骨　Humerus
5 橈骨　Radius

単純X線側面像

四肢

111

四 肢
Limbs

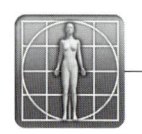

手 Hand

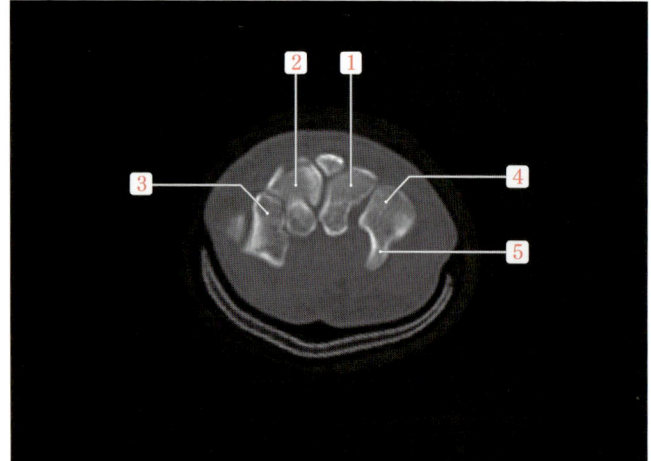

単純CT（横断像）

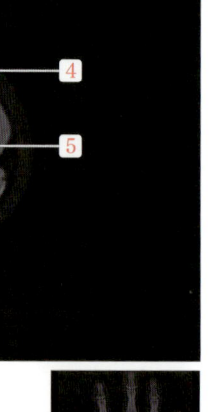

1 有頭骨　Capitate
2 小菱形骨　Trapezoid
3 大菱形骨　Trapezium
4 有鉤骨　Hamate
5 有鉤骨鉤状突起　Hook of hamate

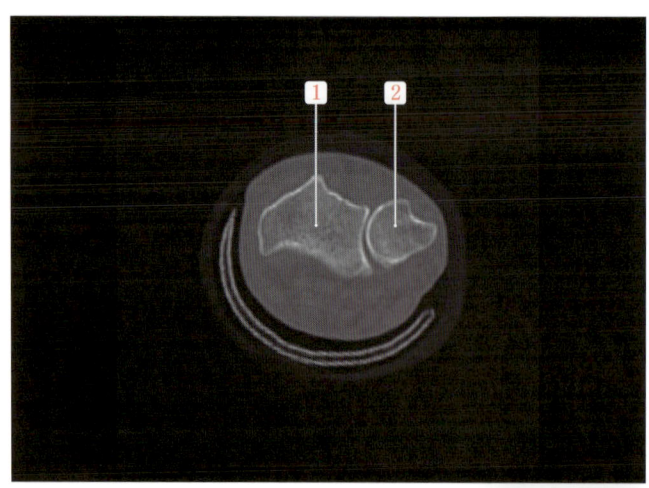

単純CT（横断像）

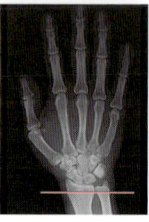

1 橈骨　Radius
2 尺骨　Ulna

● CT・MRI 解体新書

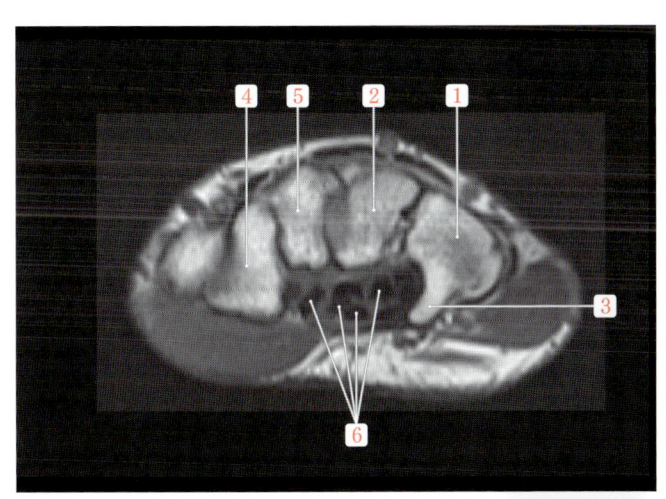

1 有鈎骨　Hamate
2 有頭骨　Capitate
3 有鈎骨鈎状突起　Hook of hamate
4 大菱形骨　Trapezium
5 小菱形骨　Trapezoid
6 屈筋腱　Flexor digitorum tendon

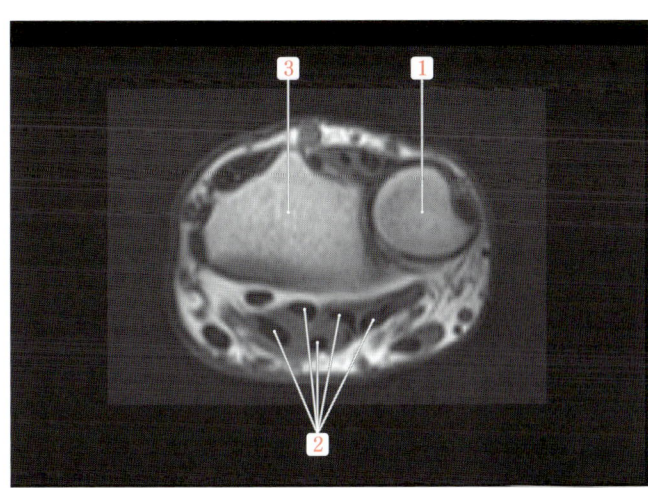

MRI T1強調像（横断像）

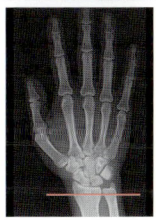

1 尺骨　Ulna
2 屈筋腱　Flexor digitorum tendon
3 橈骨　Radius

MRI T1強調像（横断像）

四肢

113

四 肢
Limbs

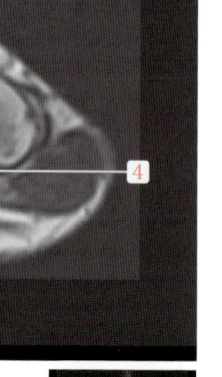

1 大菱形骨　Trapezium
2 小菱形骨　Trapezoid
3 有鈎骨　Hamate
4 有鈎骨鈎状突起　Hook of hamate
5 屈筋腱　Flexor digitorum tendon
6 有頭骨　Capitate

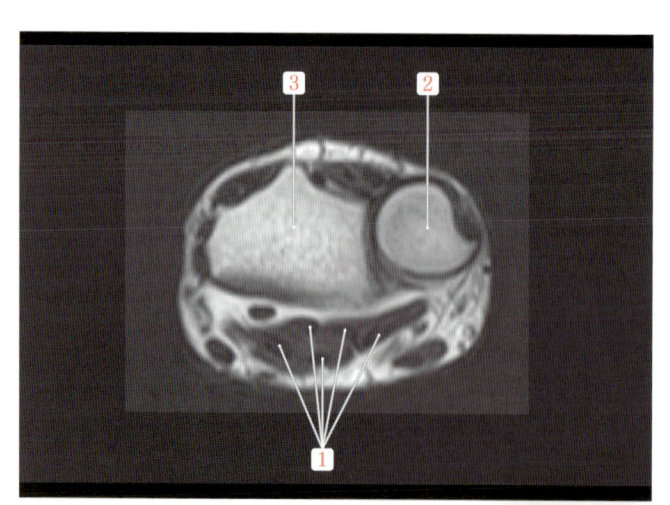

MRI T2強調像（横断像）

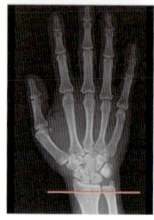

1 屈筋腱　Flexor digitorum tendon
2 尺骨　Ulna
3 橈骨　Radius

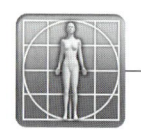

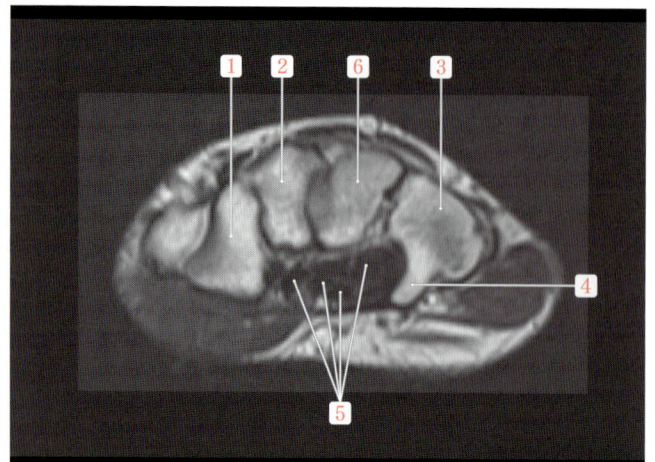

MRI T2強調像（横断像）

114

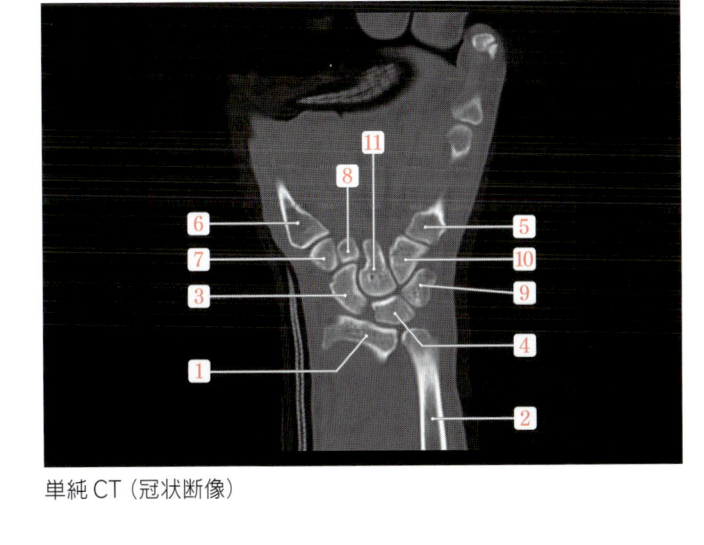

1	橈骨	Radius
2	尺骨	Ulna
3	舟状骨	Scaphoid
4	月状骨	Lunate
5	第5中手骨	Fifth metacarpal
6	第1中手骨	First metacarpal
7	大菱形骨	Trapezium
8	小菱形骨	Trapezoid
9	三角骨	Triquetrum
10	有鈎骨	Hamate
11	有頭骨	Capitate

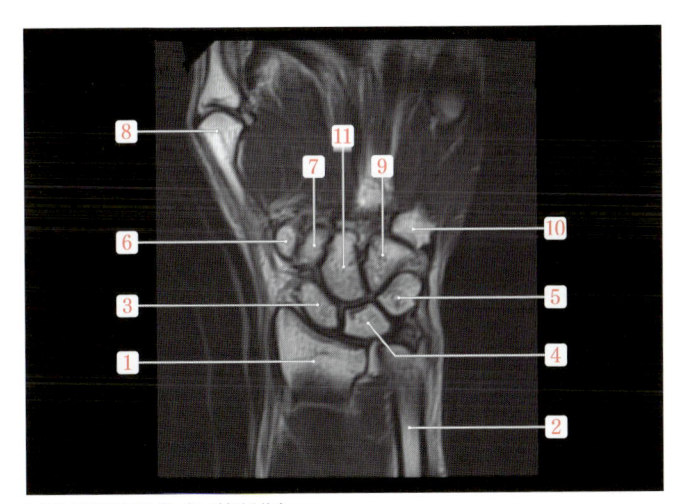

単純CT（冠状断像）

1	橈骨	Radius
2	尺骨	Ulna
3	舟状骨	Scaphoid
4	月状骨	Lunate
5	三角骨	Triquetrum
6	大菱形骨	Trapezium
7	小菱形骨	Trapezoid
8	第1中手骨	First metacarpal
9	有鈎骨	Hamate
10	第5中手骨	Fifth metacarpal
11	有頭骨	Capitate

MRI T2強調像（冠状断像）

四 肢
Limbs

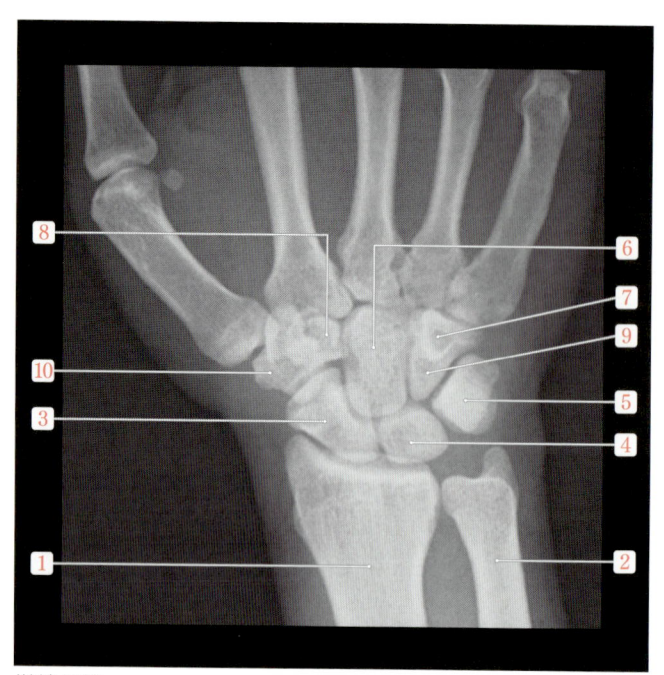

1　橈骨　Radius
2　尺骨　Ulna
3　舟状骨　Scaphoid
4　月状骨　Lunate
5　三角骨　Triquetrum
6　有頭骨　Capitate
7　有鈎骨鈎状突起　Hook of hamate
8　小菱形骨　Trapezoid
9　有鈎骨　Hamate
10　大菱形骨　Trapezium

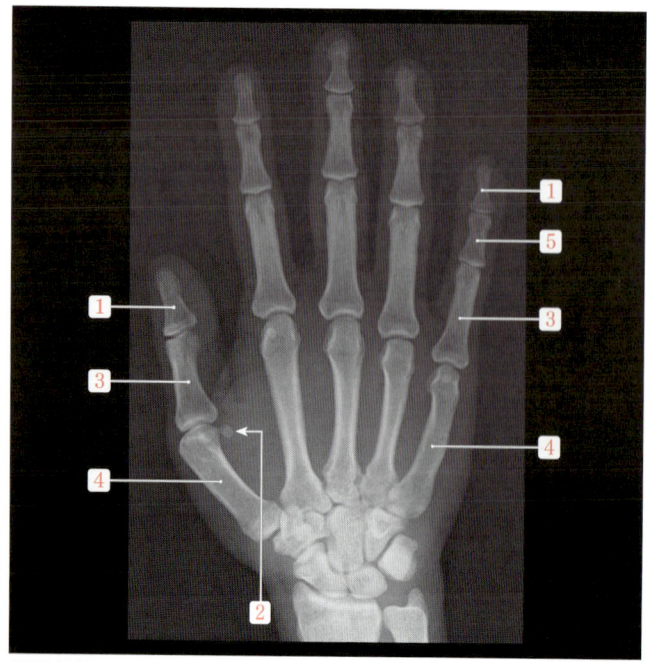

単純X線

1　末節骨　Distal phalanx
2　種子骨　Sesamoid
3　基節骨　Proximal phalanx
4　中手骨　Metacarpal
5　中節骨　Middle phalanx

単純X線

● CT・MRI 解体新書

股 Hip

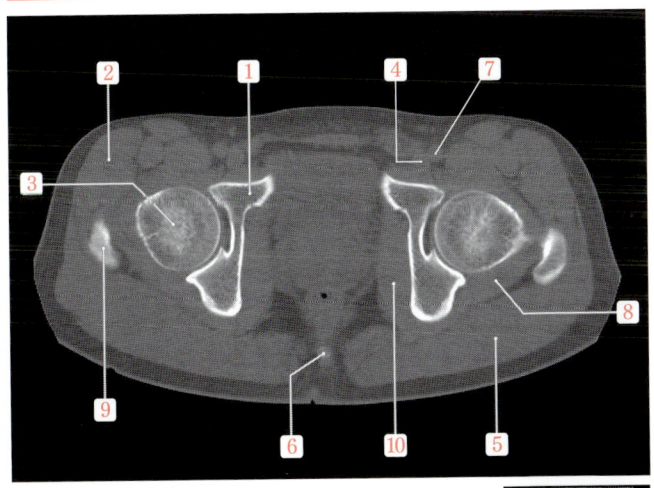

単純CT（横断像）

1 寛骨臼　Acetabulum
2 中殿筋　Gluteus medius
3 大腿骨頭　Femoral head
4 大腿静脈　Femoral vein
5 大殿筋　Gluteus maximus
6 尾骨　Coccyx
7 大腿動脈　Femoral artery
8 双子筋　Gemellus
9 大転子　Greater trochanter
10 内閉鎖筋　Internal obturator

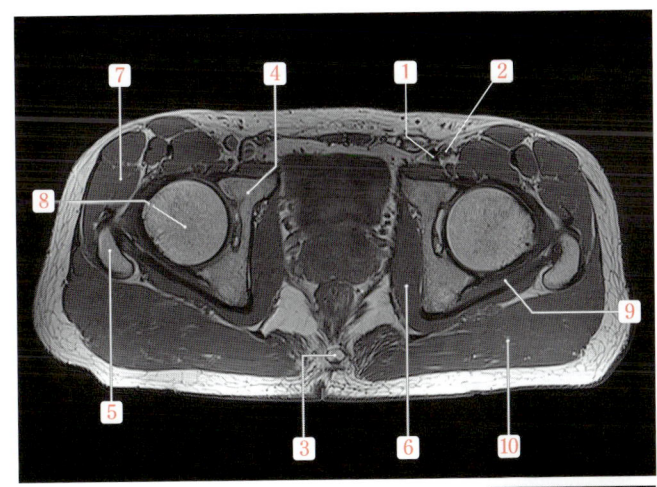

MRI T1強調像（横断像）

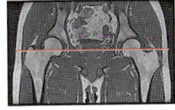

1 大腿静脈　Femoral vein
2 大腿動脈　Femoral artery
3 尾骨　Coccyx
4 寛骨臼　Acetabulum
5 大転子　Greater trochanter
6 内閉鎖筋　Internal obturator
7 中殿筋　Gluteus medius
8 大腿骨頭　Femoral head
9 双子筋　Gemellus
10 大殿筋　Gluteus maximus

四肢

117

四肢
Limbs

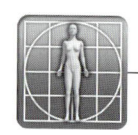

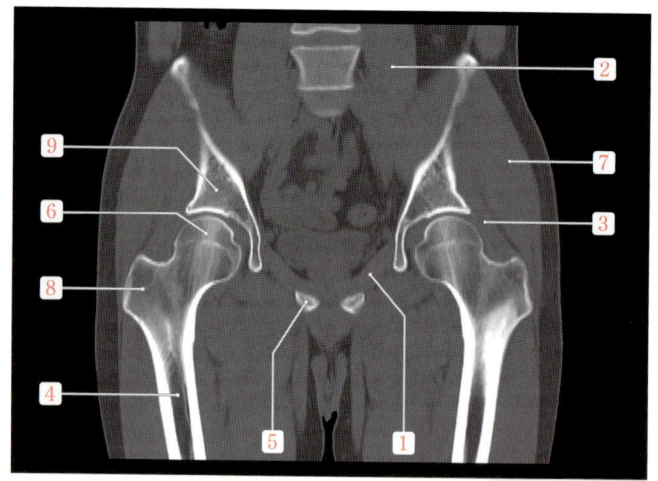

単純 CT（冠状断像）

1 内閉鎖筋　Internal obturator
2 腸腰筋　Iliopsoas
3 小殿筋　Gluteus minimus
4 大腿骨幹　Femoral shaft
5 恥骨　Pubis
6 大腿骨頭　Femoral head
7 中殿筋　Gluteus medius
8 大転子　Greater trochanter
9 寛骨臼　Acetabulum

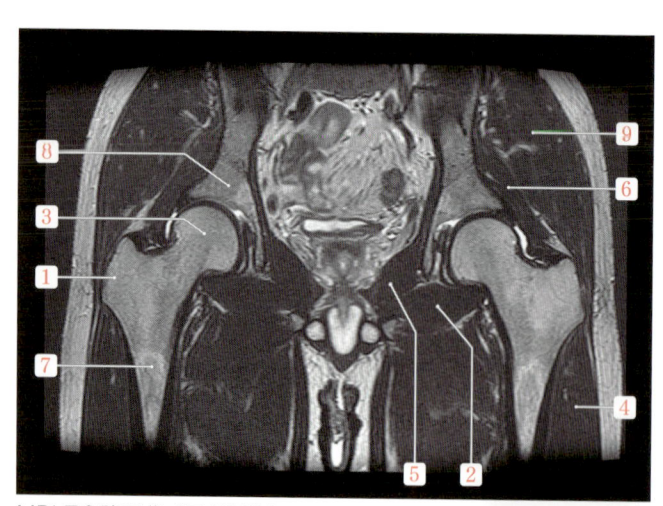

MRI T2 強調像（冠状断像）

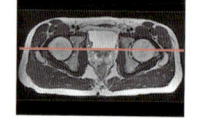

1 大転子　Greater trochanter
2 外閉鎖筋　External obturator
3 大腿骨頭　Femoral head
4 外側広筋　Vastus lateralis
5 内閉鎖筋　Internal obturator
6 小殿筋　Gluteus minimus
7 大腿骨幹　Femoral shaft
8 寛骨臼　Acetabulum
9 中殿筋　Gluteus medius

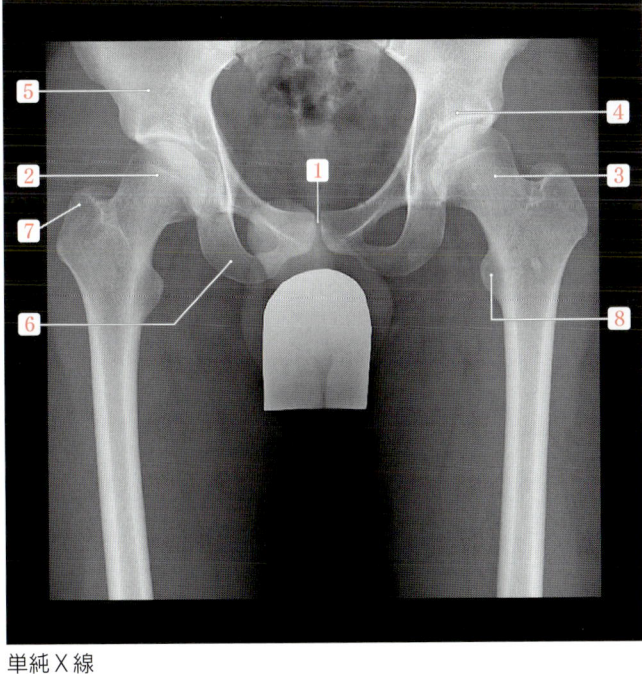

1　恥骨結合　Pubic symphysis
2　大腿骨頭　Femoral head
3　大腿骨頸　Femoral neck
4　寛骨臼蓋　Acetabular roof
5　腸骨　Ilium
6　坐骨結節　Ischial tuberosity
7　大転子　Greater trochanter
8　小転子　Lesser trochanter

単純X線

四 肢
Limbs

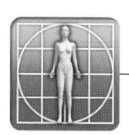

膝 Knee

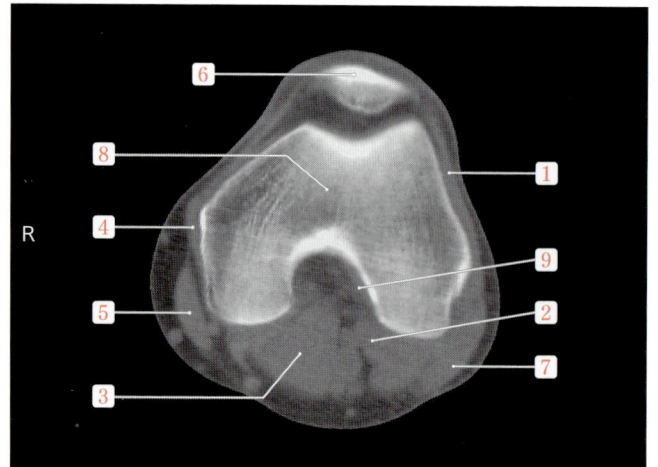

単純CT（横断像）

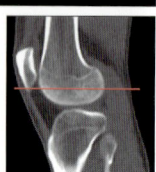

1 腸脛靱帯　Iliotibial band
2 腓腹筋外側頭　Lateral head of gastrocnemius
3 腓腹筋内側頭　Medial head of gastrocnemius
4 内側側副靱帯　Medial collateral ligament
5 縫工筋　Sartorius
6 膝蓋骨　Patella
7 大腿二頭筋　Biceps femoris
8 大腿骨　Femur
9 前十字靱帯　Anterior cruciate ligament

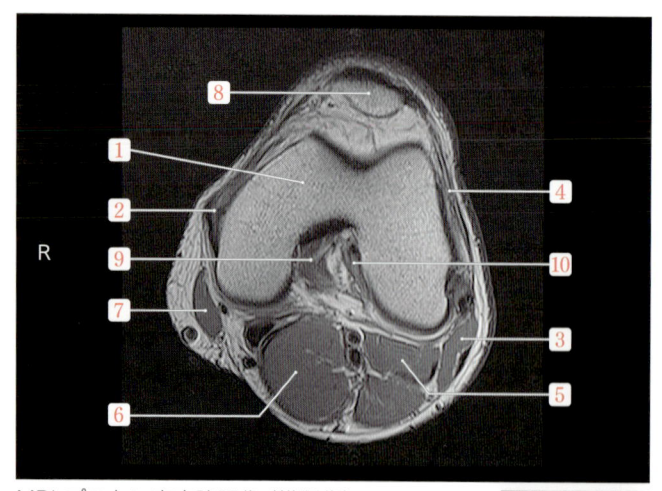

MRI プロトン密度強調像（横断像）

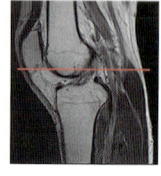

1 大腿骨　Femur
2 内側側副靱帯　Medial collateral ligament
3 大腿二頭筋　Biceps femoris
4 腸脛靱帯　Iliotibial band
5 腓腹筋外側頭　Lateral head of gastrocnemius
6 腓腹筋内側頭　Medial head of gastrocnemius
7 縫工筋　Sartorius
8 膝蓋骨　Patella
9 後十字靱帯　Posterior cruciate ligament
10 前十字靱帯　Anterior cruciate ligament

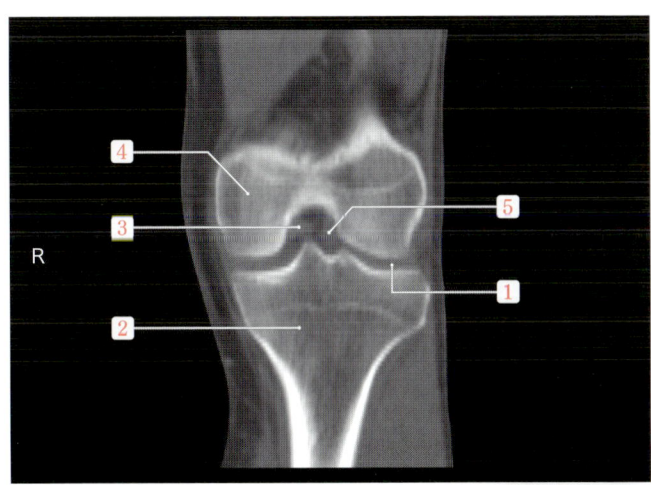

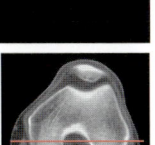

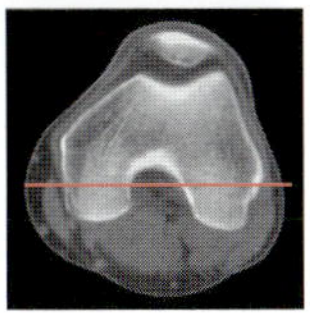

1 外側半月板　Lateral meniscus
2 脛骨　Tibia
3 後十字靱帯　Posterior cruciate ligament
4 大腿骨　Femur
5 前十字靱帯　Anterior cruciate ligament

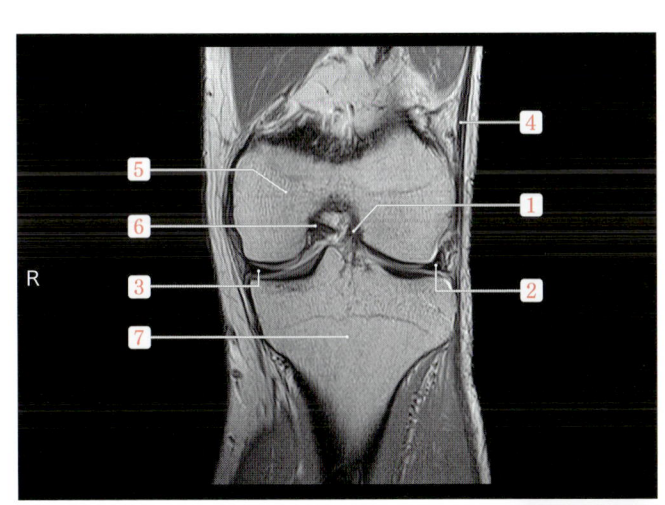

単純CT（冠状断像）

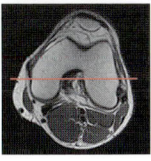

1 前十字靱帯　Anterior cruciate ligament
2 外側半月板　Lateral meniscus
3 内側半月板　Medial meniscus
4 腸脛靱帯　Iliotibial band
5 大腿骨　Femur
6 後十字靱帯　Posterior cruciate ligament
7 脛骨　Tibia

MRIプロトン密度強調像（冠状断像）

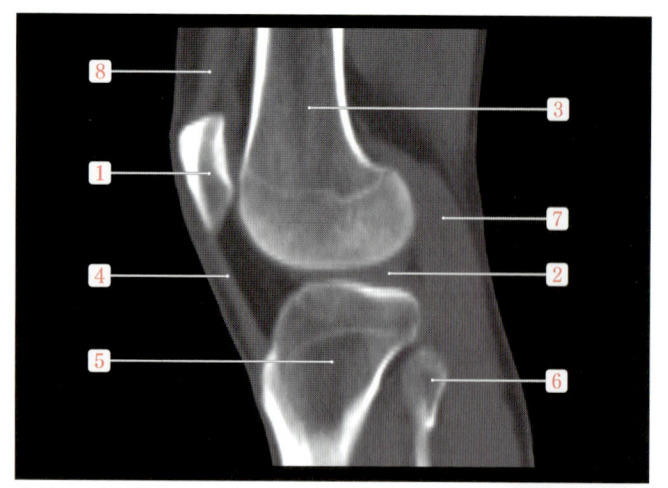

四 肢
Limbs

1 膝蓋骨　Patella
2 外側半月板　Lateral meniscus
3 大腿骨　Femur
4 膝蓋靱帯　Patellar ligament
5 脛骨　Tibia
6 腓骨　Fibula
7 腓腹筋外側頭　Lateral head of gastrocnemius
8 大腿四頭筋腱　Quadriceps femoris tendon

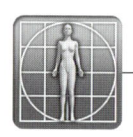

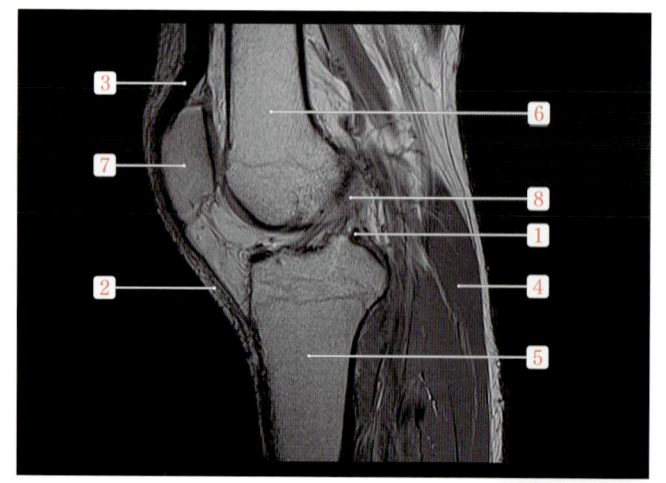

単純CT（矢状断像）

1 後十字靱帯　Posterior cruciate ligament
2 膝蓋靱帯　Patellar ligament
3 大腿四頭筋腱　Quadriceps femoris tendon
4 腓腹筋内側頭　Medial head of gastrocnemius
5 脛骨　Tibia
6 大腿骨　Femur
7 膝蓋骨　Patella
8 前十字靱帯　Anterior cruciate ligament

MRIプロトン密度強調像（矢状断像）

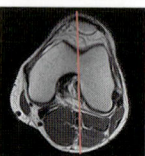

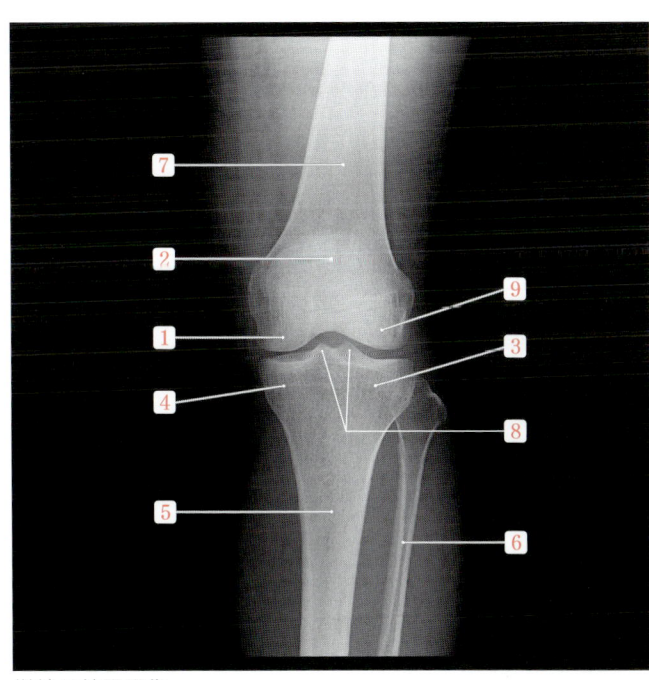

1 大腿骨内側上顆
　Medial femoral epicondyle
2 膝蓋骨　Patella
3 脛骨外側顆　Lateral tibial condyle
4 脛骨内側顆　Medial tibial condyle
5 脛骨　Tibia
6 腓骨　Fibula
7 大腿骨　Femur
8 内側および外側顆間結節
　Medial and lateral intercondylar tubercles
9 大腿骨外側上顆
　Lateral femoral epicondyle

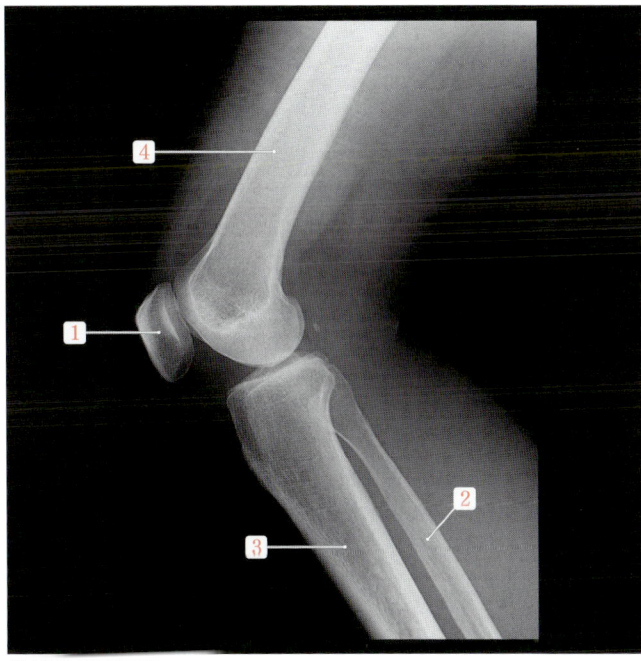

単純X線正面像

1 膝蓋骨　Patella
2 腓骨　Fibula
3 脛骨　Tibia
4 大腿骨　Femur

単純X線側面像

四肢
Limbs

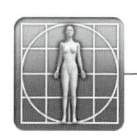

■ 足 Foot

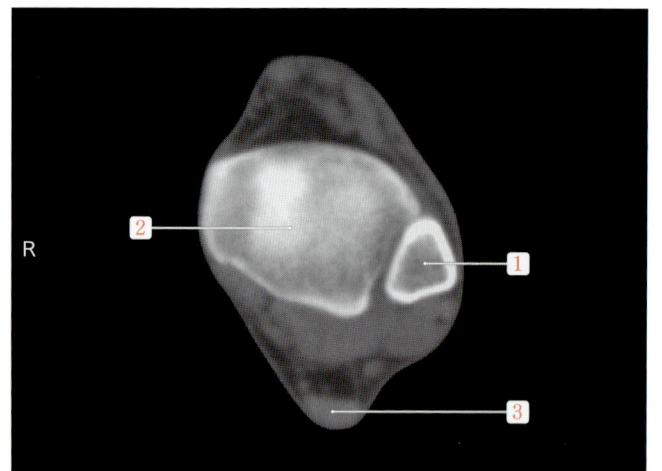

単純CT（横断像）

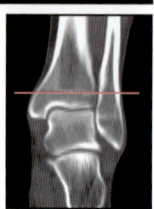

1 腓骨　Fibula
2 脛骨　Tibia
3 アキレス腱　Achilles tendon

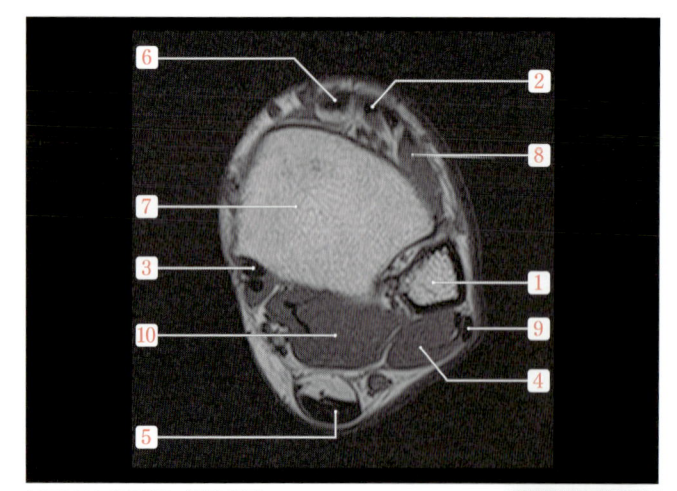

MRI T1強調像（横断像）

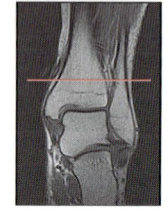

1 腓骨　Fibula
2 長母趾伸筋腱
　 Extensor hallucis longus tendon
3 後脛骨筋腱　Tibialis posterior tendon
4 長腓骨筋　Peroneus longus
5 アキレス腱　Achilles tendon
6 前脛骨筋腱　Tibialis anterior tendon
7 脛骨　Tibia
8 長趾伸筋
　 Extensor digitorum longus
9 短腓骨筋腱　Peroneus brevis tendon
10 長母趾屈筋
　 Flexor hallucis longus

単純CT（冠状断像）

1 脛骨　Tibia
2 外果　Lateral malleolus
3 踵骨　Calcaneus
4 腓骨　Fibula
5 距骨　Talus

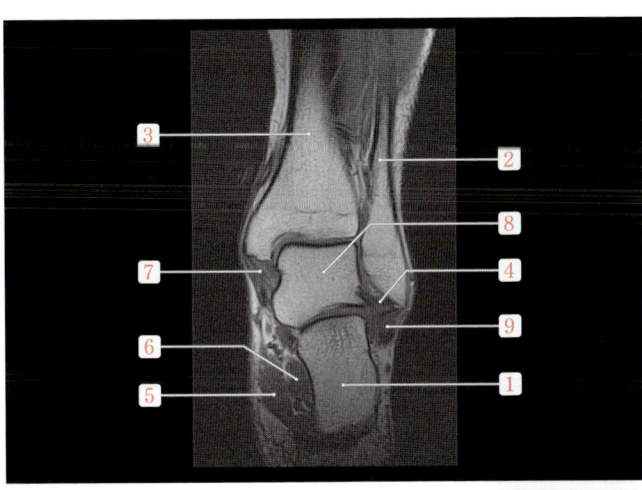

MRI T1強調像（冠状断像）

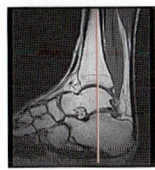

1 踵骨　Calcaneus
2 腓骨　Fibula
3 脛骨　Tibia
4 後距腓靱帯　Posterior talofibular ligament
5 母趾外転筋　Abductor hallucis
6 足底方形筋　Quadratus plantae
7 三角靱帯　Deltoid ligament
8 距骨　Talus
9 踵腓靱帯　Calcaneofibular ligament

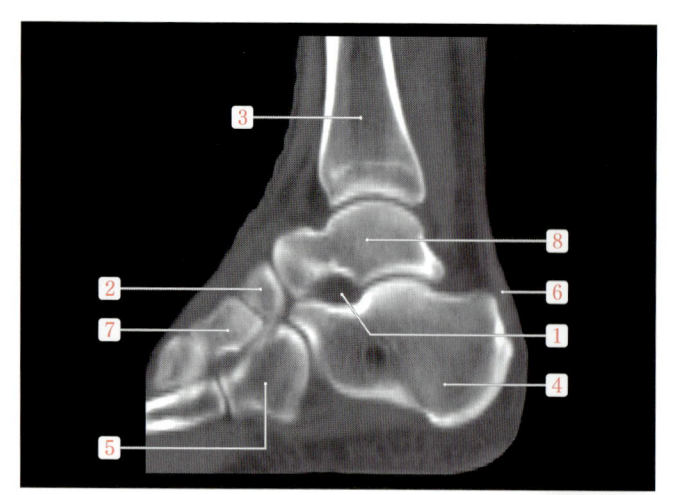

四 肢
Limbs

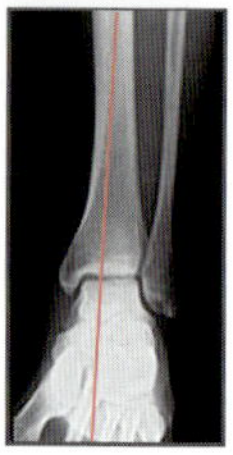

1 足根洞　Tarsal sinus
2 舟状骨　Navicular
3 脛骨　Tibia
4 踵骨　Calcaneus
5 立方骨　Cuboid
6 アキレス腱　Achilles tendon
7 中間楔状骨　Intermediate cuneiform
8 距骨　Talus

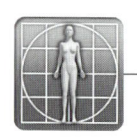

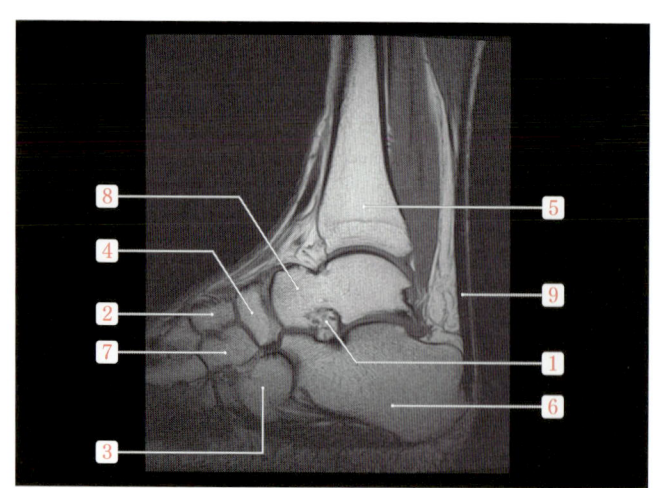

単純CT（矢状断像）

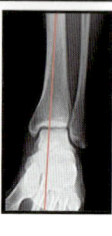

1 足根洞　Tarsal sinus
2 中間楔状骨　Intermediate cuneiform
3 立方骨　Cuboid
4 舟状骨　Navicular
5 脛骨　Tibia
6 踵骨　Calcaneus
7 外側楔状骨　Lateral cuneiform
8 距骨　Talus
9 アキレス腱　Achilles tendon

MRI T1強調像（矢状断像）

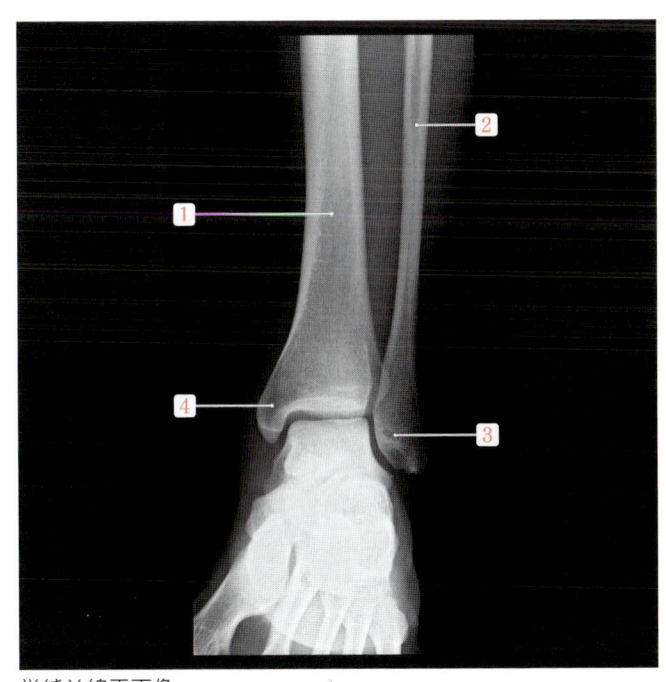

1 脛骨　Tibia
2 腓骨　Fibula
3 外果　Lateral malleolus
4 内果　Medial malleolus

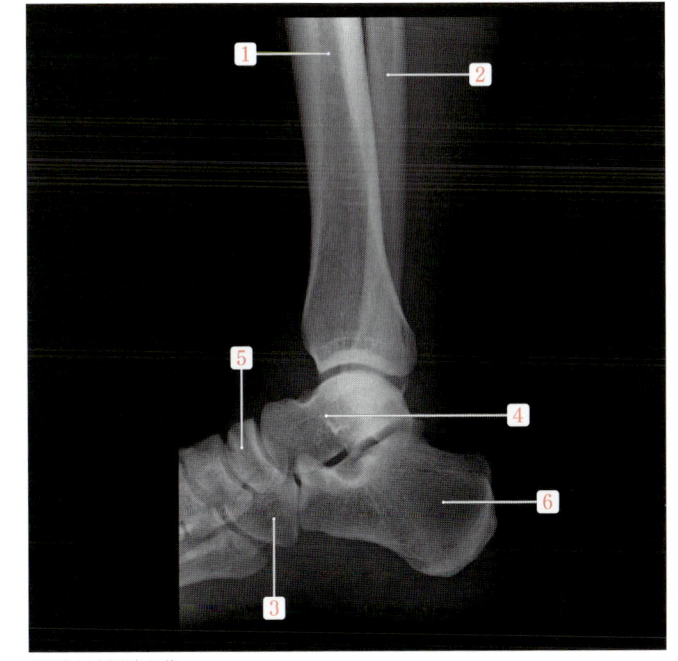

単純X線正面像

1 脛骨　Tibia
2 腓骨　Fibula
3 立方骨　Cuboid
4 距骨　Talus
5 舟状骨　Navicular
6 踵骨　Calcaneus

単純X線側面像

四肢

四 肢
Limbs

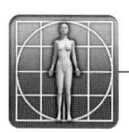

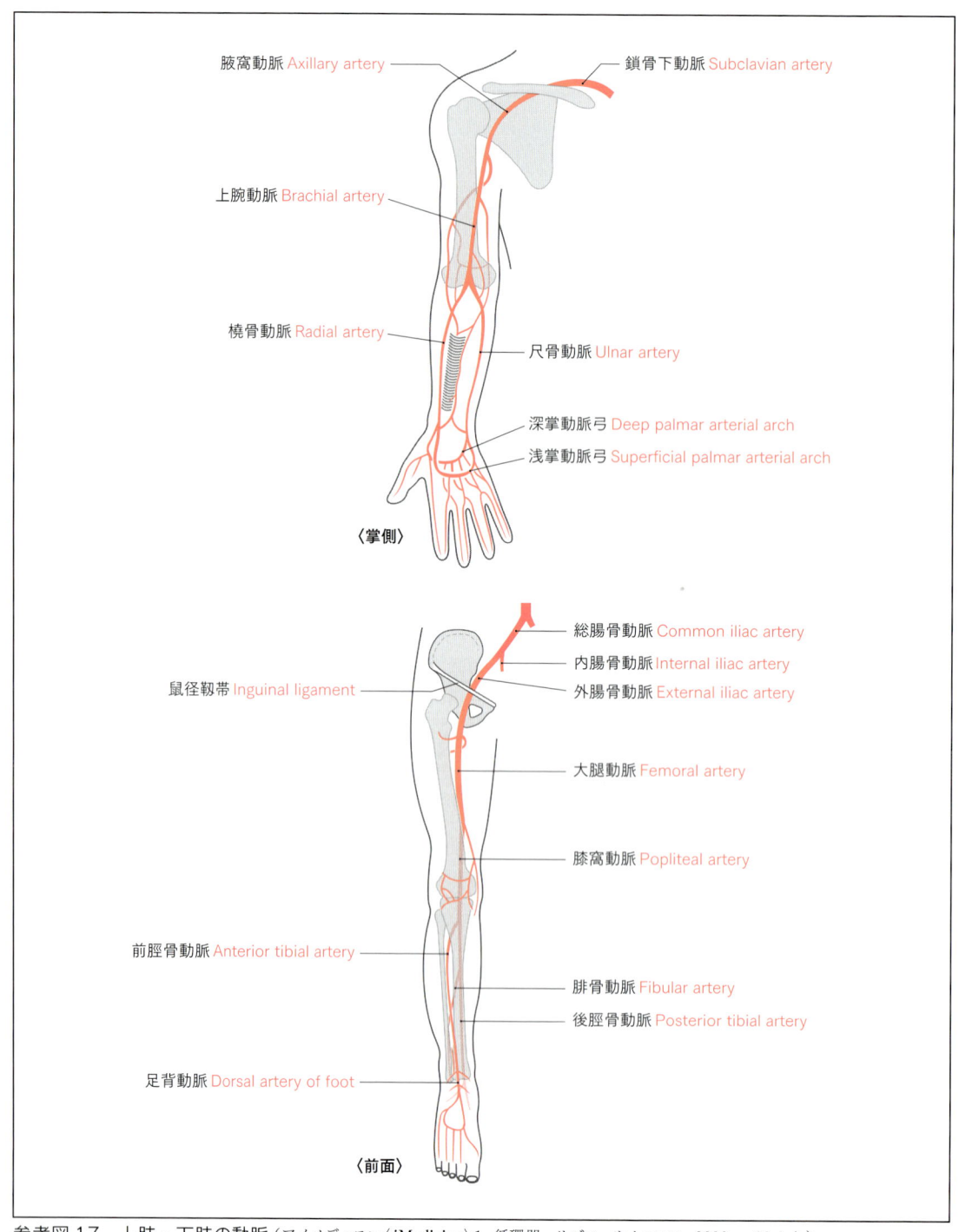

腋窩動脈 Axillary artery
鎖骨下動脈 Subclavian artery
上腕動脈 Brachial artery
橈骨動脈 Radial artery
尺骨動脈 Ulnar artery
深掌動脈弓 Deep palmar arterial arch
浅掌動脈弓 Superficial palmar arterial arch
〈掌側〉

総腸骨動脈 Common iliac artery
内腸骨動脈 Internal iliac artery
外腸骨動脈 External iliac artery
鼠径靱帯 Inguinal ligament
大腿動脈 Femoral artery
膝窩動脈 Popliteal artery
前脛骨動脈 Anterior tibial artery
腓骨動脈 Fibular artery
後脛骨動脈 Posterior tibial artery
足背動脈 Dorsal artery of foot
〈前面〉

参考図17　上肢・下肢の動脈（アイメディスン〈*i*Medicine〉1.循環器．リブロ・サイエンス，2008, p.22 より）

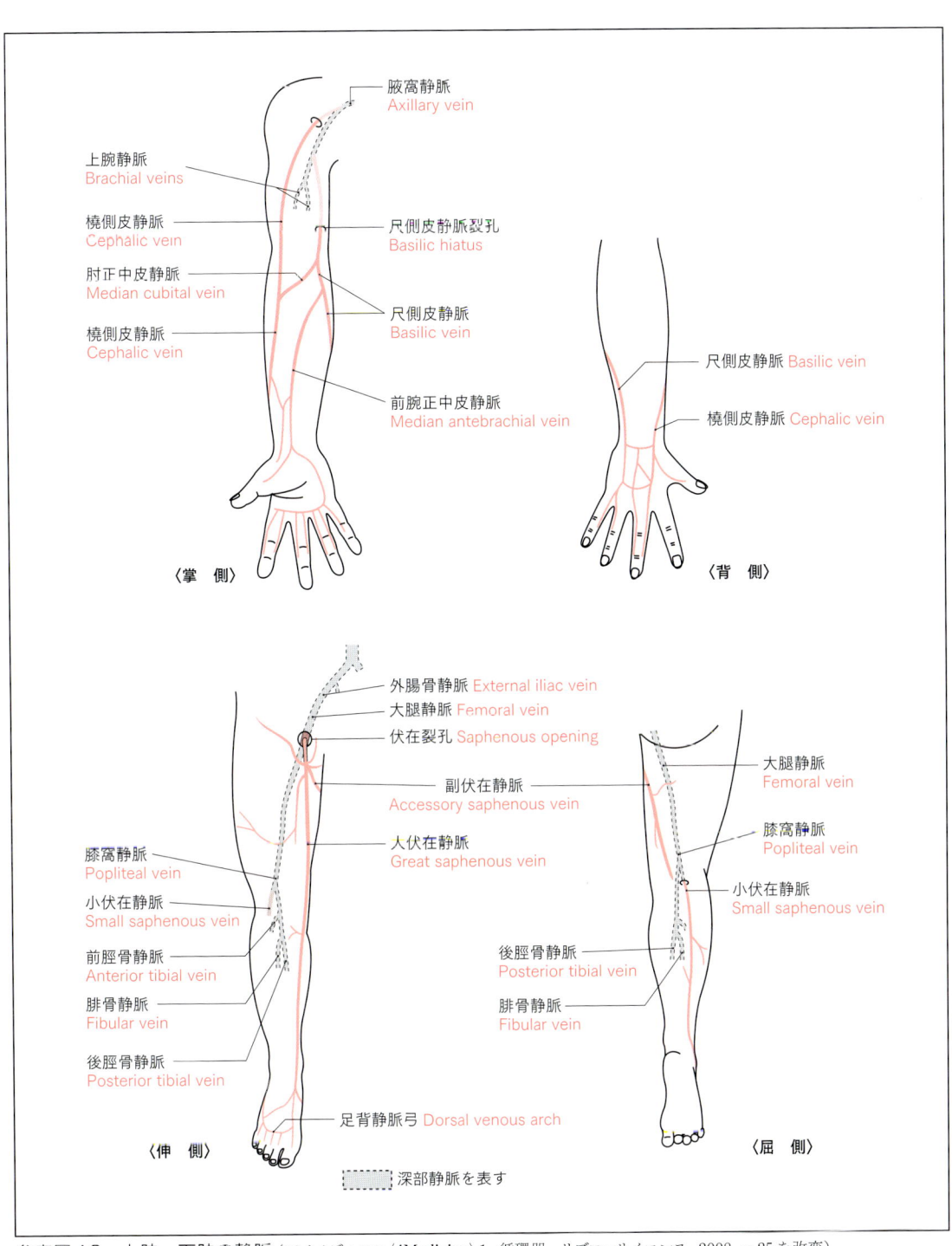

参考図18　上肢・下肢の静脈（アイメディスン〈*i*Medicine〉1. 循環器. リブロ・サイエンス, 2008, p.25を改変）

CT・MRI 解体新書

- 正常解剖 -

頭部
Head

頭頸部
Neck

脊椎
Spine

胸部
Chest

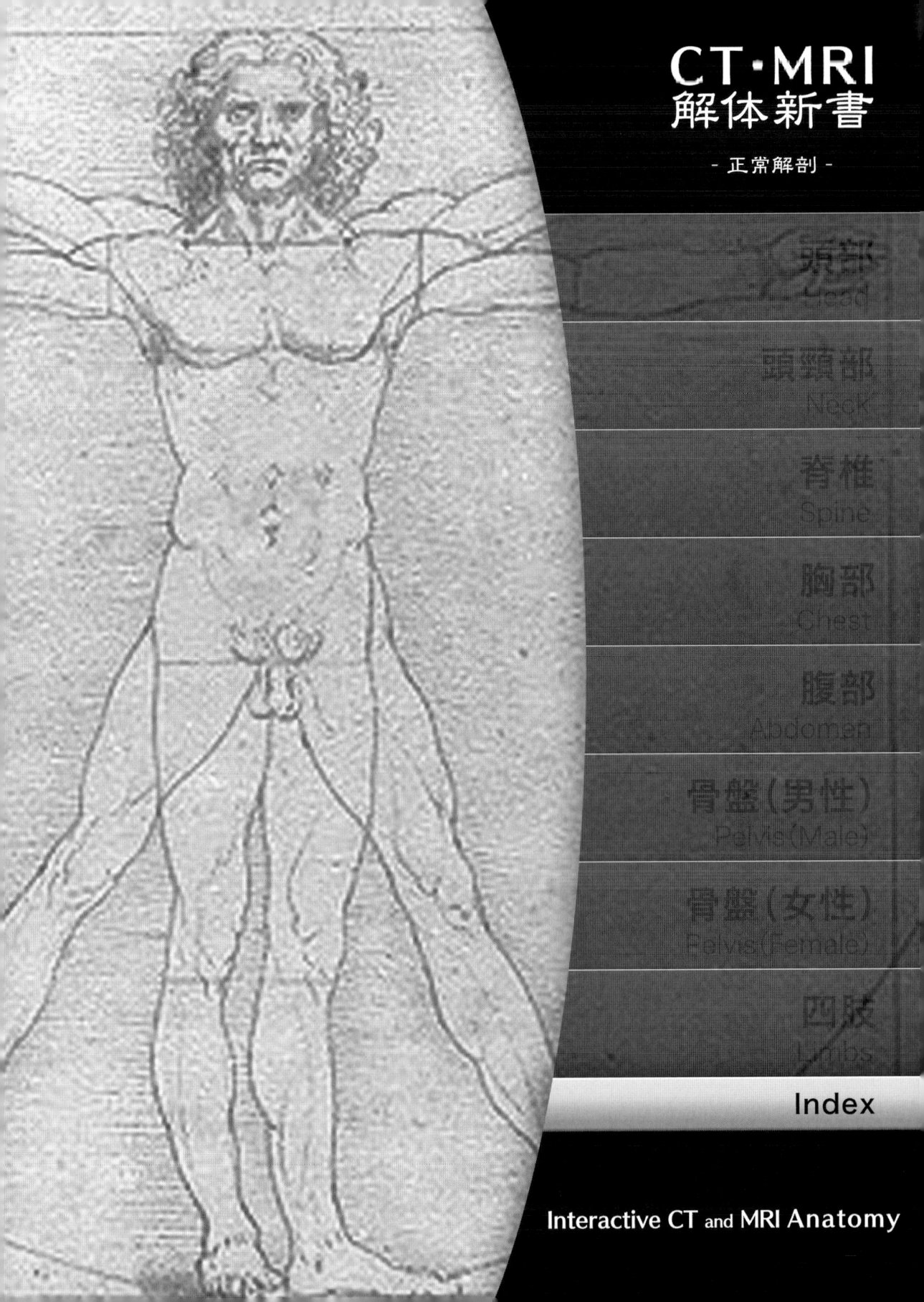

腹部
Abdomen

骨盤（男性）
Pelvis (Male)

骨盤（女性）
Pelvis (Female)

四肢
Limbs

Index

Interactive CT and MRI Anatomy

索 引
Index

"f" は図中の用語を表す。

和文索引

あ
アキレス腱　124, 126
アブミ骨　28, 29
鞍上槽　5, 9, 13
鞍背　6, 16, 17

い
胃　72-75, 79-82, 84-87, 89, 90
胃冠状静脈　88f
胃十二指腸動脈　77f, 91, 92
陰茎　96

う
ウィリス動脈輪　20f, 32f
迂回槽　5, 9, 13
烏口突起　104-107
右腎　75-77, 82, 83, 87, 88, 90
右腎静脈　75
右腎動脈　73-75
右心耳　49, 68
右心室　50, 61-65, 68
右心房　50, 61, 65
右肺
　―下葉　53-57
　―上葉　51-54
　―中葉　53-57
右肺静脈　67
右肺動脈　49, 60, 66

え
腋窩静脈　129f
腋窩動脈　128f
延髄　6, 10, 14, 16, 17

円錐枝　69

お
黄色靱帯　35-37, 39-41
横突起　35, 43, 44
横突孔　38f

か
カントリー線　78f
下顎後静脈　22, 25, 26
下顎骨　23, 26, 34
　―下顎枝　22, 25
下関節突起　35, 36, 42, 44
下丘　16, 17
下行大動脈　48-50, 60-63, 67, 72, 84
下肢の静脈　129f
下肢の動脈　128f
下膵十二指腸動脈　91f, 92
下膵動脈　77f
下垂体　9, 13, 15-17
下垂体柄　5, 9, 13, 15
下舌区　58f
下前頭回　8, 12, 15
下大静脈　50, 62, 63, 66, 70f, 72-77, 79-90
下腸間膜静脈　70f, 77f, 88f
下腸間膜動脈　70f, 92
　―の枝　92f
下直筋　30, 31
下鼻甲介　30, 31
下葉気管支　54
蝸牛　28
外果　125, 127
外頸静脈　70f
外頸動脈　26, 70f

外耳道　29
外側顆間結節　123
外側下区域（肝）　78
外側楔状骨　126
外側上顆　111
外側上区域（肝）　78
外側上葉区　58f
外側側副靱帯（肘）　109
外側直筋　30, 31
外側肺底区　58f
外側半規管　28
外側半月板　121, 122
外側広筋　118
外側翼突筋　22, 25
外腸骨静脈　70f, 129f
外腸骨動脈　70f, 96f, 128f
外閉鎖筋　96, 99, 101, 118
回結腸動脈　91f, 92
回腸　91f
回腸動脈　91f
顎下腺　23, 26
顎二腹筋　23, 26
眼窩　6
寛骨臼　117, 118
寛骨臼蓋　96, 119
肝区域　78f
肝静脈　70f, 78f
　中―　63, 72, 73, 79, 83f, 84
　左―　63, 72, 79, 83f, 84
　右―　63, 72, 73, 79, 83f, 84
肝臓　63, 67, 72, 74-76, 79, 80, 82-85, 87-90
　―の区域　78
関節唇　107
　後―　105
　前―　105

環椎　38f
　—横靭帯　38f
　—外側塊　34f
　—後弓　34,37,39,40
　—前弓　34,37,40,42
冠動脈　68,69,70f
　左—　69
　右—　68,69
　—セグメント（AHAによる）
　　69f

き

キヌタ骨　28
気管　27,46-48,51,52,59,65,66
奇静脈　48-50,70f
奇静脈弓　48
基節骨　116
脚間槽　4,9,13
距骨　125-127
橋　5,9,13,16,17
橋前槽　5,9,10,13,14,16,17
橋動脈　20f
胸骨　59-62
胸鎖乳突筋　23,24,26,27
胸神経　38f
胸椎　27,90
棘下筋　105
棘下筋腱　105
棘上筋　107
棘上筋腱　107
棘上靭帯　40,41
棘突起　35-44

く

クモ膜下腔　34,39,40
空腸　91f
空腸動脈　91f
屈筋腱　113,114

け

脛骨　121-127
　—外側顆　123
　—内側顆　123
頸神経　38f
頸髄　26
頸椎　23,24
　—椎体　26,27
月状骨　115,116
結節間溝　104,105
結腸　89
　上行—　90
結腸動脈　92f
肩甲下筋　105,106
肩甲下筋腱　105
肩甲棘　106
肩甲骨　107
　—関節窩　104-107
肩鎖関節　106,107
肩峰　106,107

こ

鼓室蓋　29
鼓室上陥凹　29
鼓膜被蓋　29
固有肝動脈　77f,83f,91f
後下区域（肝）　78
後下行枝（冠動脈）　69
後関節唇　105
後距腓靭帯　125
後脛骨筋腱　124
後脛骨静脈　129f
後脛骨動脈　128f
後交通動脈　18-20f,32f
後十字靭帯　120-122
後縦靭帯　39-41
後上区域（肝）　78
後上葉区　58f
後膵動脈　77f

後脊髄動脈　20f
後側壁枝（冠動脈）　69
後大脳動脈　18-20f,32f
後頭葉　3,5,7,11
後肺底区　58f
後半規管　28
口蓋扁桃　22,25
咬筋　22,25,34
甲状腺　27,46
甲状軟骨　24
鈎状突起（頸椎）　42
鈎状突起（尺骨）　110,111
喉頭　24
喉頭蓋　23
喉頭蓋谷　23
硬膜外脂肪　37,38,40,41
肛門　101
肛門挙筋　94,95,99,101

さ

鎖骨　104,106,107
鎖骨下静脈　70f
鎖骨下動脈　32f,70f
　左—　46,47,59,66
坐骨　94,95,98-101
　—結節　119
左腎　73-77,81-83,86-88,90
左腎静脈　74,75,81,86
左腎動脈　74,75
左心室　50,61-65,68
左心房　49,50,61,66-68
左肺
　—下葉　52-57
　—上葉　51-54
　—上葉舌区　55-57
左肺静脈　66
左肺動脈　48,66,67
三角筋　105,107
三角骨　115,116
三角靭帯　125

索引
Index

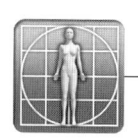

さ
三叉神経　14

し
シルビウス裂　3-5, 8, 12, 15
耳下腺　22, 25
耳管咽頭口　22, 25
子宮　98
　　― 頸部　100, 102
　　― 体部　100, 102
四丘体槽　4, 8, 12, 16, 17
視交叉　4, 8, 12, 15
視床　3, 8, 12
視床間橋　6f, 16, 17
視神経　9, 13, 16, 17, 20f, 30, 31
　　右―　13
篩骨洞　10, 14
軸椎　38
　　― 歯突起　34, 37-40, 42
膝窩静脈　129f
膝窩動脈　128f
膝蓋骨　120, 122, 123
膝蓋靱帯　122
斜台　37
尺側皮静脈　129f
　　― 裂孔　129f
尺骨　108-116
　　― 肘頭　108, 111
尺骨神経　108
尺骨動脈　128f
主気管支
　　左―　48, 53, 60, 67
　　右―　48, 53, 60, 67
主膵管　89
種子骨　116
舟状骨(手)　115, 116
舟状骨(足)　126, 127
十二指腸　75, 76, 82, 87, 90
十二指腸水平脚　75
松果体　3
上 - 下葉区　58f

上顎骨　22, 25
上顎洞　10, 14, 22, 25, 30, 31
上関節突起　35, 36, 42, 44
上丘　16, 17
上行結腸　90
上行大動脈　48, 49, 60, 61, 65, 68
上肢の静脈　129f
上肢の動脈　128f
上矢状静脈洞　2, 3, 8, 12
上斜筋　30, 31
上小脳動脈　19, 20f
上膵十二指腸動脈　92f
上舌区　58f
上前頭回　8, 12, 15
上大静脈　48, 49, 59-61, 66, 70f
上腸間膜静脈　70f, 75-77f, 82, 87, 88f
上腸間膜動脈　70f, 74-77, 81, 82, 86, 87, 91f, 92f
　　― の枝　92f
上直筋　30, 31
上直腸動脈　92f
上腕骨　108-111
　　― 滑車　110, 111
　　― 小頭　110, 111
　　― 頭　104-107
上腕静脈　129f
上腕動脈　128f
上腕二頭筋長頭腱　105, 107
小結節　104, 105
小腸の血管支配　91f
小殿筋　118
小転子　119
小脳テント　5
小脳脚　5, 10, 14
小脳橋角槽　6
小脳虫部　4, 8, 9, 12, 13
小脳半球　5, 6, 10, 14, 16, 17
小伏在静脈　129f
小葉間裂　53, 54

小菱形骨　112-116
踵骨　125-127
踵腓靱帯　125
静脈洞交会　4
食道　27, 46-50, 59-63
食道胃移行部　72
食道静脈　88f
心室中隔　50, 62-64
心房回旋枝　69
深掌動脈弓　128f
深大腿動脈　95
腎静脈　70f
　　右―　75
　　左―　74, 75, 81, 86
腎臓
　　右―　75-77, 82, 83, 87-90
　　左―　73-77, 81-83, 86-88, 90
腎動脈　70f
　　右―　73-75
　　左―　74, 75

す
膵管　89
膵臓　73-77, 80-82, 85-87, 89
　　― の脈管系　77f

せ
精索　94, 95
精嚢　94, 95
声帯　24, 27
脊髄　34, 36, 39-41
脊柱管　34, 35, 37, 38
舌　22, 25
舌骨　23, 26
前下区域(肝)　78
前下小脳動脈　20f
前関節唇　105
前脛骨筋腱　124
前脛骨静脈　129f
前脛骨動脈　128f

134

前鼓室上陥凹　28
前交通動脈　20^f, 32^f
前喉頭蓋間隙　26
前十字靱帯　120-122
前縦靱帯　39-41
前上区域（肝）　78
前上葉区　58^f
前床突起　5
前脊髄動脈　20^f, 32^f
前大脳動脈　18, 19, 32^f
前頭葉　3, 5, 7, 11
前脈絡叢動脈　20^f
前肺底区　58^f
前立腺　94, 96
　―中心域　95
　―辺縁域　95
前腕正中皮静脈　129^f
仙骨　38, 102
仙骨神経　38^f
仙腸関節　90
仙椎　90
浅掌動脈弓　128^f
浅側頭動脈　18
浅大腿動脈　95

そ

鼠径靱帯　96^f, 128^f
総肝管　83^f
総肝動脈　73, 74, 77^f, 91^f
総頸動脈　24, 26, 27, 32^f, 46, 70^f
　―左―　46, 47, 59, 66
総胆管　74, 75, 77, 81-83^f, 86, 87, 90
総腸骨静脈　70^f
総腸骨動脈　70^f, 96^f, 128^f
双子筋　117
足根洞　126
足底方形筋　125
足背静脈弓　129^f
足背動脈　128^f

側頭骨　5, 6
側頭葉　5-7, 11
側脳室　3, 6^f, 7, 11, 15
　―後角　3, 6^f
　―三角部　8, 12
　―前角　3, 4, 6^f, 8, 12

た

第1対角枝（冠動脈）　69
第1中手骨　115
第2対角枝（冠動脈）　69
第5中手骨　115
第三脳室　3, 4, 8, 12
第四脳室　5, 6^f, 9, 10, 13, 14, 16, 17
大結節　104, 105
大槽　16, 17
大腿管　96^f
大腿骨　99, 101, 120-123
　―外側上顆　123
　―幹　118
　―頸　119
　―頭　94-96, 98, 100, 117-119
　―内側上顆　123
大腿四頭筋腱　122
大腿静脈　70^f, 94, 95, 98, 101, 117
大腿神経　96^f
大腿動脈　94, 95, 98, 101, 117, 128^f
　深―　95
　浅―　95
大腿二頭筋　120
大腸の血管支配　92^f
大殿筋　94, 98-100, 117
大転子　117-119
大動脈
　下行―　48-50, 60-63, 67, 72, 84
　上行―　48, 49, 60, 61, 65, 68

　腹部―　66, 72-77, 79-88, 90
大動脈弓　32^f, 48, 59, 66, 67
大動脈弁　49, 61
大脳鎌　2, 3, 7, 11
大脳脚　8, 12
大脳縦裂　4, 7, 11
大伏在静脈　129^f
大葉間裂
　左―　52-57
　右―　53-57
大腰筋　36, 90
大菱形骨　112-116
帯状回　16, 17
帯状溝　16, 17
短胃動脈　91^f
胆管　83^f
胆嚢　74-76, 82, 83^f, 87, 89
胆嚢動脈　91^f
短腓骨筋腱　124

ち

恥骨　98, 102, 118
恥骨筋　99, 101
恥骨結合　99, 101, 119
腟　101, 102
中間気管支幹　53, 54
中間楔状骨　126
中肝静脈　63, 72, 73, 78^f, 79, 83^f, 84
中手骨　116
　第1―　115
　第5―　115
中心管　6^f
中心溝　2, 7, 11
中心後回　2, 7, 11
中心前回　2, 7, 11
中節骨　116
中前頭回　8, 12, 15
中大脳動脈　13, 18-20^f, 32^f
中殿筋　117, 118

索引
Index

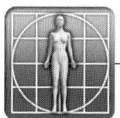

中脳　4, 8, 12
中脳水道　4-6^f, 9, 13, 16, 17
虫垂動脈　91^f, 92^f
肘頭　110
腸脛靱帯　120, 121
腸骨　90, 100, 119
腸腰筋　100, 118
蝶形骨洞　10, 14, 16, 17
長趾伸筋　124
長腓骨筋　124
長母趾屈筋　124
長母趾伸筋腱　124
直腸　94, 95, 98, 100, 102
直腸周囲腔　94, 95
直動脈　91^f

つ

ツチ骨　28, 29
椎間関節　35, 36, 42
　　　―柱　42
椎間孔　43, 44
椎間板　35, 39-41
椎間板腔　37, 38
椎弓　36
椎弓根　35, 36, 42-44
椎骨動脈　18-20^f, 26, 32^f, 70^f
椎体　35-44
椎体静脈　39, 41

と

トルコ鞍　5
洞結節動脈　69
橈骨　109-116
　　　―頭　108, 110, 111
橈骨動脈　128^f
橈側皮静脈　129^f
頭頂後頭溝　16, 17
透明中隔　3
鈍縁枝　69

な

内果　127
内胸動脈　70^f
内頸静脈　24, 26, 27, 46, 70^f
内頸動脈　9, 13, 15, 18-20^f, 26, 32^f, 70^f
内耳道　10, 14, 28
内側顆間結節　123
内側区域（肝）　78
内側上顆　111
内側側副靱帯（肘）　109
内側側副靱帯（膝）　120
内側中葉区　58^f
内側直筋　30, 31
内側肺底区　58^f
内側半月板　121
内側翼突筋　34
内腸骨静脈　70^f
内腸骨動脈　70^f, 128^f
内閉鎖筋　94-96, 98, 99, 101, 117, 118
内包　3, 12, 15

に

乳頭体　8, 12
乳突洞　28
尿道　101

の

脳室の構造　6^f
脳脊髄液　34, 39-41
脳底動脈　10, 14, 18-20^f, 32^f
脳梁　3, 7, 8, 11, 12, 15
　　　―膝部　16, 17
　　　―体部　16, 17
　　　―膨大部　8, 12, 16, 17

は

馬尾　36
肺区域　58^f
肺静脈
　　　右―　67
　　　左―　66
肺尖区　58^f
肺尖後区　58^f
肺動脈　64-66
　　　右―　49, 60, 66
　　　左―　48, 66, 67
　　　―幹　49, 60, 64, 65, 68
肺動脈弁　49, 61
半月板
　　　外側―　121, 122
　　　内側―　121
半卵円中心　2

ひ

鼻甲介
　　　下―　30, 31
腓骨　122-125, 127
腓骨静脈　129^f
腓骨動脈　128^f
腓腹筋外側頭　120, 122
腓腹筋内側頭　120, 122
尾骨　94, 95, 98, 117
尾骨神経　38^f
尾状核　12, 15
尾状葉　78
脾静脈　70^f, 73-75, 77^f, 81, 88^f
脾臓　67, 72-75, 79-82, 84-87, 89, 90
脾動脈　73, 77^f, 91^f
鼻中隔　10, 14, 22, 25
披裂喉頭蓋ヒダ　26
披裂軟骨　24, 27
左下葉気管支　54
左肝静脈　63, 72, 78^f, 79, 83^f, 84

左肝動脈　91^f
左冠動脈　69
　　— 回旋枝　68, 69
　　— 主幹部　68, 69
　　— 前下行枝　68, 69
左鎖骨下動脈　46, 47, 59, 66
左主気管支　48, 53, 60, 67
左総頸動脈　46, 47, 59, 66
左大葉間裂　52-57
左副腎　73, 85
左卵巣　98, 100
左腕頭静脈　46, 47, 59

ふ

プルサック腔　29
腹腔動脈　70^f, 73, 77^f, 80, 85, 91^f
　　— の枝　91^f
腹部大動脈　66, 70^f, 72-77^f, 79-88, 90
伏在裂孔　129^f
副腎
　　左 —　73, 85
　　右 —　73, 74, 80, 85
副伏在静脈　129^f

へ

辺縁動脈　92^f

ほ

母趾外転筋　125
膀胱　94-96, 98, 100, 102

縫工筋　120
房室枝　69
放線冠　3

ま

末節骨　116

み

右肝静脈　63, 72, 73, 78^f, 79, 83^f, 84
右肝動脈　91^f
右冠動脈　68, 69
右視神経　13
右主気管支　48, 53, 60, 67
右大葉間裂　53-57
右副腎　73, 74, 80, 85
右卵巣　98, 100
右腕頭静脈　46, 47, 59, 65
脈絡叢　8, 12

も

モンロー孔　6^f, 8, 12
門脈　77^f, 78^f, 83^f, 88^f, 90
　　— 右枝　73, 81
　　— 左枝　72, 73, 80, 85
　　— 本幹　74, 81, 85, 86

ゆ

有鈎骨　112-116
　　— 鈎状突起　112-114, 116
有頭骨　112-116

よ

腰神経　38^f
腰椎　90

ら

卵巣
　　左 —　98, 100
　　右 —　98, 100

り

梨状陥凹　23, 24, 26
梨状筋　100
立方骨　126, 127

れ

レンズ核　3, 8, 12, 15

ろ

ローゼンミューラー窩　22, 25
肋椎関節　35, 36
肋骨　27

わ

腕頭静脈　70^f
　　左 —　46, 47, 59
　　右 —　46, 47, 59, 65
腕頭動脈　32^f, 46, 47, 59, 65, 70^f

索引
Index

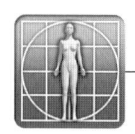

欧文索引

A

Abdominal aorta 66, 70^f, 72-77^f, 79-88, 90
Abductor hallucis 125
Accessory saphenous vein 129^f
Acetabular roof 96, 119
Acetabulum 117, 118
Achilles tendon 124, 126
Acromioclavicular joint 106, 107
Acromion 106, 107
Adrenal gland 73, 74, 80, 85
　Left ─ 73, 85
　Right ─ 73, 74, 80, 85
Ambient cistern 5, 9, 13
Anterior arch of atlas 34, 37, 40, 42
Anterior basal segment 58^f
Anterior cerebral artery 18-20^f, 32^f
Anterior choroidal artery 20^f
Anterior clinoid process 5
Anterior communicating artery 20^f, 32^f
Anterior cruciate ligament 120-122
Anterior epitympanic recess 28
Anterior horn of lateral ventricle 3, 4, 6^f, 8, 12
Anterior inferior cerebellar artery 20^f
Anterior labrum 105
Anterior longitudinal ligament 39-41
Anterior segment 58^f
Anterior spinal artery 20^f, 32^f
Anterior tibial artery 128^f
Anterior tibial vein 129^f
Anus 101
Aorta
　Abdominal ─ 66, 70^f, 72-77^f, 79-88, 90
　Descending ─ 48-50, 60-63, 67, 72, 84
Aortic arch 32^f, 48, 59, 66, 67
Aortic valve 49, 61
Apical segment 58^f
Apicoposterior segment 58^f
Appendicular artery 91^f, 92^f
Aqueduct 4-6^f, 9, 13, 16, 17
Arteries
　Anterior cerebral 18-20^f, 32^f
　Anterior choroidal 20^f
　Anterior communicating 20^f, 32^f
　Anterior inferior cerebellar 20^f
　Anterior spinal 20^f, 32^f
　A-V node 69^f
　Axillary 128^f
　Basilar 10, 14, 18-20^f, 32^f
　Brachial 128^f
　Brachiocephalic 32^f, 46, 47, 59, 65, 70^f
　Celiac 70^f, 73, 77^f, 80, 85
　Colic 92^f
　Common carotid 24, 26, 27, 32^f, 46, 70^f
　Common hepatic 73, 74, 77^f, 83^f, 91^f
　Common iliac 70^f, 96^f, 128^f
　Cystic 91^f
　Deep femoral 95
　Dorsal pancreatic 77^f
　External carotid 70^f
　External iliac 70^f, 96^f, 128^f
　Femoral 94, 95, 98, 101, 117, 128^f
　Fibular 128^f
　Gastroduodenal 77^f, 91^f, 92^f
　Ileal 91^f
　Iliocolic 91^f, 92^f
　Inferior mesenteric 70^f, 92^f
　Inferior pancreatic 77^f
　Internal carotid 9, 13, 15, 18-20^f, 26, 32^f, 70^f
　Internal iliac 70^f, 128^f
　Internal thoracic 70^f
　Jejunal 91^f
　Left anterior descending coronary (LAD) 68, 69
　Left circumflex coronary (LCX) 68, 69
　Left common carotid 46, 47, 59, 66
　Left coronary (LCA) 69
　Left gastric 77^f, 91^f
　Left hepatic 91^f
　Left pulmonary 48, 66, 67
　Left renal 74, 75
　Left subclavian 46, 47, 59, 66
　Middle cerebral 13, 18-20^f, 32^f
　Popliteal 128^f
　Posterior cerebral 18-20^f, 32^f
　Posterior communicating 18-20^f, 32^f
　Posterior inferior cerebellar 20^f
　Posterior tibial 128^f
　Proper hepatic 77^f, 91^f
　Pulmonary 64-66
　Radial 128^f
　Renal 70^f
　Rectal 92^f
　Right coronary (RCA) 68, 69
　Right hepatic 91^f
　Right pulmonary 49, 60, 66
　Right renal 73-75
　Short gastric 91^f
　Sinus node 69
　Splenic 73, 77^f, 91^f

138

Subclavian 32f, 70f, 128f
Superficial femoral 95
Superficial temporal 18
Superior cerebellar 19, 20f
Superior mesenteric 70f, 74-77f, 81, 82, 86, 87, 91f
Ulnar 128f
Vertebral 20f, 70f
Articular pillar 42
Ary-epiglottic fold 26
Arytenoid cartilage 24, 27
Ascending aorta 48, 49, 60, 61, 65, 68
Ascending colon 90
Atlas 38f
   Anterior arch of — 34, 37, 40, 42
   Lateral mass of — 34
   Posterior arch of — 34, 37, 39, 40
   Transverse ligament of — 38f
Atrial circumflex branch (AC) 69f
A-V node artery (AV) 69f
Axillary artery 128f
Axillary vein 129f
Axis 38f
Azygos arch 48
Azygos vein 48-50, 70f

B

Basilar artery 10, 14, 18-20f, 32f
Basilic hiatus 129f
Basilic vein 129f
Basivertebral vein 39, 41
Biceps femoris 120
Body of corpus callosum 16, 17
Brachial artery 128f
Brachial vein 129f
Brachiocephalic artery 32f, 46, 47, 59, 65, 70f

Brachiocephalic vein 46, 47, 59, 70f
Bronchus 48, 53, 60, 67

C

Calcaneofibular ligament 125
Calcaneus 125-127
Cantlie 線 78f
Capitate 112-116
Capitulum 110, 111
Cauda equina 36
Caudate lobe 78
Caudate nucleus 12, 15
Celiac artery 70f, 73, 77f, 80, 85
Central canal 6f
Central sulcus 2, 7, 11
Centrum semiovale 2
Cephalic vein 129f
Cerebellar hemisphere 5, 6, 10, 14, 16, 17
Cerebellar peduncle 5, 10, 14
Cerebellar tentorium 5
Cerebellar vermis 4, 8, 9, 12, 13
Cerebellopontine angle cistern 6
Cerebral peduncle 8, 12
Cerebrospinal fluid 34, 39-41
Cervical nerve 38f
Cervical spinal cord 26
Cervical vertebra 23
Cervical vertebral body 24, 26, 27
Choroid plexus 8, 12
Cingulate gyrus 16, 17
Cingulate sulcus 16, 17
Cisterna magna 16, 17
Clavicle 104, 106, 107
Clivus 37
Coccygeal nerve 38f
Coccyx 94, 95, 98, 117
Cochlea 28
Colic artery 92f

Colon 89, 90
Common bile duct 74, 75, 77f, 81-83f, 86, 87, 90
Common carotid artery 24, 26, 27, 32f, 46, 70f
Common hepatic artery 73, 74, 77f, 91f
Common hepatic duct 83f
Common iliac artery 70f, 96f, 128f
Common iliac vein 70f
Conus arteriosus 49, 61
Conus branch (CB) 69f
Coracoid process 104-107
Corona radiata 3
Coronoid process 110, 111
Corpus callosum 3, 7, 8, 11, 12, 15
   Body of — 16, 17
   Genu of — 16, 17
   Splenium of — 8, 12, 16, 17
Costovertebral joint 35, 36
Cuboid 126, 127
Cystic artery 91f

D

Deep femoral artery 95
Deep palmar arterial arch 128f
Deltoid ligament 125
Deltoid 105, 107
Descending aorta 48-50, 60-63, 67, 72, 84
Diagonal branch 69
Digastric 23, 26
Distal phalanx 116
Dorsal artery of foot 128f
Dorsal pancreatic artery 77f
Dorsal venous arch 129f
Dorsum sellae 6, 16, 17
Duodenum 75, 76, 82, 87, 90
   Horizontal part of — 75

索引
Index

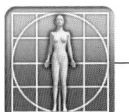

E

Epidural fat 37, 38, 40, 41
Epiglottis 23
Epitympanic recess 29
Esophageal vein 89^f
Esophagogastric junction 72
Esophagus 27, 46-50, 59-63
Ethmoidal sinus 10, 14
Extensor digitorum longus 124
Extensor hallucis longus tendon 124
External auditory canal 29
External carotid artery 26, 70^f
External iliac artery 70^f, 96^f, 128^f
External iliac vein 70^f
External jugular vein 70^f, 129^f
External obturator 96, 99, 101, 118

F

Facet joint 35, 36
Falx cerebri 2, 3, 7, 11
Femoral artery 94, 95, 98, 101, 117, 128^f
Femoral canal 96^f
Femoral head 94-96, 98, 100, 117-119
Femoral neck 119
Femoral nerve 96^f
Femoral shaft 118
Femoral vein 70^f, 94-96^f, 98, 101, 117
Femur 99, 101, 120-123
Fibula 122-125, 127
Fibular artery 128^f
Fibular vein 129^f
First diagonal branch 69
Flexor digitorum tendon 113, 114
Flexor hallucis longus 124

Foramen of Luschka 6^f
Foramen of Magendie 6^f
Foramen of Monro 6^f, 8, 12
Fourth ventricle 5, 6^f, 9, 10, 13, 14, 16, 17
Frontal lobe 3, 5, 7, 11

G

Gallbladder 74-76, 82, 87, 89
Gastric coronary vein 88^f
Gastroduodenal artery 77^f, 91^f, 92^f
Gemellus 117
Genu of corpus callosum 16, 17
Glenoid cavity of scapula 104-107
Gluteus maximus 94, 98-100, 117
Gluteus medius 117, 118
Gluteus minimus 118
Great saphenous vein 129^f
Greater trochanter 117-119
Greater tubercle 104, 105

H

Hamate 112-116
　Hook of ― 112-114, 116
Head of radius 108, 110, 111
Hepatic vein 70^f, 78^f, 83^f
　Left ― 63, 72, 78^f, 79, 83^f, 84
　Middle ― 63, 72, 73, 79, 84
　Right ― 63, 72, 73, 78^f, 79, 83^f, 84
Hook of hamate 112-114, 116
Horizontal part of duodenum 75
Humeral head 104-107
Humerus 108-111
Hyoid bone 23, 26

I

Ibialis anterior tendon 124
Ileal artery 91^f
Iliocolic artery 91^f, 92^f

Iliopsoas 100, 118
Iliotibial band 120, 121
Ilium 90, 91^f, 100, 119
Incus 28
Inferior articular process 35, 36, 42, 44
Inferior colliculus 16, 17
Inferior frontal gyrus 8, 12, 15
Inferior lingular segment 58^f
Inferior mesenteric artery 70^f, 92^f
Inferior mesenteric vein 70^f, 77^f, 88^f
Inferior nasal concha 30, 31
Inferior pancreatic artery 77^f
Inferior rectus 30, 31
Inferior vena cava 50, 62, 63, 66, 70^f, 72-77, 79-88, 90
Infraspinatus 105
Infraspinatus tendon 105
Inguinal ligament 96^f, 128^f
Intermediate cuneiform 126
Internal auditory canal 10, 14, 28
Internal capsule 3, 12, 15
Internal carotid artery 9, 13, 15, 18-20^f, 26, 32^f, 70^f
Internal iliac artery 70^f, 128^f
Internal iliac vein 70^f
Internal jugular vein 24, 26, 27, 46, 70^f
Internal obturator 94-96, 98, 99, 101, 117, 118
Internal thoracic artery 70^f
Interpeduncular cistern 4, 9, 13
Interthalamic adhesion 6^f, 16, 17
Intertubercular sulcus 104, 105
Interventricular septum 50, 62-64
Intervertebral disc 35, 39-41
Intervertebral disc space 37, 38
Intervertebral foramen 43, 44
Intervertebral joint 42

Ischial tuberosity   119
Ischium   94, 95, 98-101

J

Jejunum   91f
Jejunal artery   91f

K

Kidney
　　Left —   73-77, 81-83, 86-88, 90
　　Right —   75-77, 82, 83, 87, 88, 90

L

Labrum   107
　　Anterior —   105
　　Posterior —   105
LAD   68, 69
Larynx   24
Lateral basal segment   58f
Lateral collateral ligament   109
Lateral cuneiform   126
Lateral epicondyle   111
Lateral femoral epicondyle   123
Lateral head of gastrocnemius   120, 122
Lateral intercondylar tubercle   123
Lateral malleolus   125, 127
Lateral mass of atlas   34
Lateral meniscus   121, 122
Lateral pterygoid   22, 25
Lateral rectus   30, 31
Lateral segment   58f
Lateral semicircular canal   28
Lateral tibial condyle   123
Lateral ventricle   3, 6f, 7, 11, 15
　　Anterior horn of —   3, 4, 8, 12
　　Inferior horn of —   6f
　　Posterior horn of —   3, 6f

Trigone of —   8, 12
LCA   69
LCX   68, 69
Left adrenal gland   73, 85
Left anterior descending coronary artery (LAD)   68, 69
Left atrium   49, 50, 61, 66-68
Left brachiocephalic vein   46, 47, 59
Left circumflex coronary artery (LCX)   68, 69
Left common carotid artery   46, 47, 59, 66
Left coronary artery (LCA)   69
Left coronary artery main stem (LMT)   68, 69
Left gastric artery   77f
Left gastro-epiploic artery   91f
Left hepatic artery   91f
Left hepatic vein   63, 72, 78f, 79, 83f, 84
Left inferior lobar bronchus   54
Left kidney   73-77, 81-83, 86-88, 90
Left lateral inferior segment   78
Left lateral superior segment   78
Left lung   52-57
　　Lower lobe of —   52-57
　　Upper lobe of —   51-54
Left main bronchus   48, 53, 60, 67
Left major fissure   52-57
Left medial segment   78
Left ovary   98, 100
Left portal vein   72, 73, 80, 85
Left pulmonary artery   48, 66, 67
Left pulmonary vein   66
Left renal artery   74, 75
Left renal vein   74, 75, 81, 86
Left subclavian artery   46, 47, 59, 66, 70f

Left ventricle   50, 61-65, 68
Lentiform nucleus   3, 8, 12, 15
Lesser trochanter   119
Lesser tubercle   104, 105
Levator ani   94, 95, 99, 101
Lingular segment   55-57
Liver   63, 67, 72, 74, 76, 79, 80, 82-85, 87-90
LMT   68, 69
Lobar bronchus   54
Longitudinal fissure   4, 7, 11
Long head of biceps brachii tendon   105, 107
Lower lobe of left lung   52-57
Lower lobe of right lung   53-57
Lumbar nerve   38f
Lumbar vertebra   90
Lunate   115, 116
Lung
　　Left —   52-57
　　Right —   53-57
Luschka 孔   6f

M

Magendie 孔   6f
Main bronchus
　　Left —   48, 53, 60, 67
　　Right —   48, 53, 60, 67
Main pancreatic duct   89
Main portal vein   74, 81, 85, 86
Major fissure
　　Left —   52-57
　　Right —   53-57
Malleus   28, 29
Mammillary body   8, 12, 20f
Mandible   23, 26, 34
Marginal artery   92f
Masseter   22, 25, 34
Mastoid antrum   28
Maxilla   22, 25

索引
Index

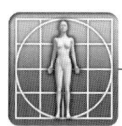

Maxillary sinus 10, 14, 22, 25, 30, 31
Medial basal segment 58f
Medial intercondylar tubercle 123
Medial collateral ligament 109, 120
Medial epicondyle 111
Medial femoral epicondyle 123
Medial head of gastrocnemius 120, 122
Medial malleolus 127
Medial meniscus 121
Medial pterygoid 34
Medial rectus 30, 31
Medial segment 58f
Medial tibial condyle 123
Median antebrachial vein 129f
Medulla oblongata 6, 10, 14, 16, 17
Mesencephalon 4, 8, 12
Metacarpal 115, 116
Middle cerebral artery 13, 18-20f, 32f
Middle frontal gyrus 8, 12, 15
Middle hepatic vein 63, 72, 73, 78f, 79, 83f, 84
Middle lobe of right lung 53-57
Middle phalanx 116
Minor fissure 53, 54
Monro 孔 6f, 8, 12
Muscles
    Abductor hallucis 125
    Biceps femoris 120
    Deltoid 105, 107
    Extensor digitorum longus 124
    External obturator 96, 99, 101, 118
    Flexor hallucis longus 124
    Gemellus 117
    Gluteus maximus 94, 98-100, 117

    Gluteus medius 117, 118
    Gluteus minimus 118
    Iliopsoas 100, 118
    Infraspinatus 105
    Internal obturator 94-96, 98, 99, 101, 117, 118
    Levator ani 94, 95, 99, 101
    Masseter 22, 25
    Medial pterygoid 34
    Pectineus 99, 101
    Peroneus longus 124
    Piriformis 100
    Psoas major 36, 90
    Quadratus plantae 125
    Sartorius 120
    Subscapularis 105, 106
    Supraspinatus 107
    Vastus lateralis 118

N
Nasal concha 30, 31
Nasal septum 10, 14, 22, 25
Navicular 126, 127

O
Obtuse marginal branch (OM) 69f
Occipital lobe 3, 5, 7, 11
Odontoid process 34, 37-40, 42
Olecranon 108, 110, 111
Optic chiasm 4, 8, 12, 15
Optic nerve 9, 13, 16, 17, 20f, 30, 31
  Right — 13
Orbit 6
Ovary
  Left — 98, 100
  Right — 98, 100

P
Palatine tonsil 22, 25
Pancreas 73-76, 80-82, 85-87, 89
Pancreatic duct 89
Parieto-occipital sulcus 16, 17
Parotid gland 22, 25
Patella 120, 122, 123
Patellar ligament 122
Pectineus 99, 101
Pedicle 35, 36, 42-44
Penis 96
Perirectal space 94, 95
Peroneus brevis tendon 124
Peroneus longus 124
Pharyngeal orifice of eustachian tube 22, 25
Pineal body 3
Piriform fossa 23, 24, 26
Piriformis 100
Pituitary gland 9, 13, 15-17
Pituitary stalk 5, 9, 15
Pons 5, 9, 13, 16, 17
Pontine arteries 20f
Popliteal artery 128f
Popliteal vein 128f
Portal vein 77f, 78f, 83f, 90
  Left — 72, 73, 80, 85
  Main — 74, 81, 85, 86
  Right — 73, 81
Postcentral gyrus 2, 7, 11
Posterior arch of atlas 34, 37, 39, 40
Posterior basal segment 58f
Posterior cerebral artery 18-20f, 32f
Posterior communicating artery 18-20f, 32f
Posterior cruciate ligament 120-122

Posterior descending branch (PD)　69
Posterior horn of lateral ventricle　3, 6f
Posterior inferior cerebellar artery　20f
Posterior labrum　105
Posterior longitudinal ligament　39-41
Posterior segment　58f
Posterior semicircular canal　28
Posterior spinal artery　20f
Posterior tibial artery　128f
Posterior tibial vein　129f
Posterior talofibular ligament　125
Posterolateral branch (PL)　69
Precentral gyrus　2, 7, 11
Pre-epiglottic space　26
Prepontine cistern　5, 9, 10, 13, 14, 16, 17
Proper hepatic artery　77f, 83f, 91f
Prostate　94, 96
　Central zone　95
　Peripheral zone　95
Proximal phalanx　116
Prussak's space　29
Psoas major　36, 90
Pubic symphysis　99, 101, 119
Pubis　98, 102, 118
Pulmonary artery　64-66
Pulmonary trunk　49, 60, 64, 65, 68
Pulmonary valve　49, 61

Q

Quadratus plantae　125
Quadriceps femoris tendon　122
Quadrigeminal cistern　4, 8, 12, 16, 17

R

Radial artery　128f
Radius　109-116
　Head of —　108, 110, 111
Ramus of mandible　22, 25
RCA　68, 69
Rectum　94, 95, 98, 100, 102
Renal artery　70f
Renal vein　70f
Retromandibular vein　22, 25, 26
Rib　27
Right adrenal gland　73, 74, 80, 85
Right anterior inferior segment　78
Right anterior superior segment　78
Right atrium　50, 61, 65
Right auricle　49, 68
Right brachiocephalic vein　46, 47, 59, 65
Right coronary artery (RCA)　68, 69
Right gastro-epiploic artery　91f
Right hepatic artery　91f
Right hepatic vein　63, 72, 73, 78f, 79, 83f, 84
Right kidney　75-77, 82, 83, 87, 88, 90
Right lung　53-57
　Lower lobe of —　53-57
　Middle lobe of —　53-57
　Upper lobe of —　51-54
Right main bronchus　48, 53, 60, 67
Right major fissure　53-57
Right optic nerve　13
Right ovary　98, 100
Right portal vein　73, 81
Right posterior inferior segment　78
Right posterior superior segment　78

Right pulmonary artery　49, 60, 66
Right pulmonary vein　67
Right renal artery　73-75
Right renal vein　75
Right ventricle　50, 61-65, 68
Rosenmüller's fossa　22, 25

S

S状結腸動脈　92f
Sacral nerve　38f
Sacral vertebra　90
Sacro-iliac joint　90
Sacrum　38, 102
Saphenous opening　129f
Sartorius　120
Scaphoid　115, 116
Scapula　107
　Glenoid cavity of —　104-107
Scapular spine　106
Scutum　29
Second diagonal branch　69
Sella turcica　5
Seminal vesicle　94, 95
Septum pellucidum　3
Sesamoid　116
Short gastric artery　91
Sigmoid artery　92f
Sinus confluence　4
Sinus node artery (SN)　69
Small saphenous vein　129f
Spermatic cord　94, 95
Sphenoidal sinus　10, 14, 16, 17
Spinal canal　34, 35, 37, 38
Spinal cord　34, 36, 39-41
Spinous process　35-44
Spleen　67, 72-75, 79-82, 84-87, 89, 90
Splenic artery　73, 77f, 91f
Splenic vein　70f, 73-75, 77f, 81, 88f

索 引
Index

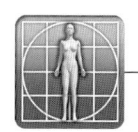

Splenium of corpus callosum 8, 12, 16, 17
Stapes 28, 29
Sternocleidomastoid 23, 24, 26, 27
Sternum 59-62
Stomach 72-75, 79-82, 84-87, 89, 90
Straight arteries 91f
Subarachnoid space 34, 39, 40
Subclavian artery 32f, 46, 47, 59, 66, 70f, 128f
Subclavian vein 70f
Submandibular gland 23, 26
Subscapularis 105, 106
Subscapularis tendon 105
Superficial femoral artery 95
Superficial palmar arterial arch 128f
Superficial temporal artery 18
Superior articular process 35, 36, 42, 44
Superior cerebellar artery 19, 20f
Superior colliculus 16, 17
Superior frontal gyrus 8, 12, 15
Superior lingular segment 58f
Superior mesenteric artery 70f, 74-77f, 81, 82, 86, 87, 91f
Superior mesenteric vein 70f, 75-77f, 82, 87, 88f
Superior oblique 30, 31
Superior pancreaticoduodenal artery 92f
Superior rectal artery 92f
Superior rectus 30, 31
Superior sagittal sinus 2, 3, 8, 12
Superior segment 58f
Superior vena cava 48, 49, 59-61, 66, 70f
Suprasellar cistern 5, 9, 13

Supraspinatus 107
Supraspinatus tendon 107
Supraspinous ligament 40, 41
Sylvian fissure 3-5, 8, 12, 15

T
Talus 125-127
Tarsal sinus 126
Tegmen tympani 29
Temporal bone 5, 6
Temporal lobe 5, 6, 7, 11
Thalamus 3, 8, 12
Third ventricle 3, 4, 6f, 8, 12
Thoracic nerve 38f
Thoracic vertebra 27, 90
Thyroid cartilage 24
Thyroid gland 27, 46
Tibia 121-127
Tibial vein 129f
Tibialis posterior tendon 124
Tongue 22, 25
Trachea 27, 46-48, 51, 52, 59, 65, 66
Transverse foramen 38f
Transverse ligament of atlas 38f
Transverse process 35, 43, 44
Trapezium 112-116
Trapezoid 112-116
Trigeminal nerve 14
Trigone of lateral ventricle 8, 12
Triquetrum 115, 116
Trochlea 110, 111
Truncus intermedius 53, 54

U
Ulna 108-116
Ulnar artery 128f
Ulnar nerve 108
Uncinate process 42
Upper lobe of left lung 51-54

Upper lobe of right lung 51-54
Urethra 101
Urinary bladder 94-96, 98, 100, 102
Uterine body 100, 102
Uterine cervix 100, 102
Uterus 98

V
Vagina 101, 102
Vallecula epiglottica 23
Vastus lateralis 118
Veins
    Axillary 129f
    Azygos 48-50, 70f
    Basilic 129f
    Basivertebral 39, 41
    Brachial 129f
    Brachiocephalic 46, 47, 59, 65, 70f
    Cephalic 129f
    Common iliac 70f
    Esophageal 88f
    External iliac 70f
    External jugular 70f
    External iliac 129f
    Femoral 70f, 94, 95, 98, 101, 117
    Gastric coronary 88f
    Hepatic 63, 70f, 72, 73, 78f, 79, 83f, 84
    Inferior mesenteric 70f, 77f, 88f
    Internal iliac 70f
    Internal jugular 24, 26, 27, 46, 70f
    Left hepatic 63, 72, 79, 84
    Left pulmonary 66
    Left renal 74, 75, 81, 86
    Main portal 74, 81, 85, 86
    Middle hepatic 63, 72, 73, 79, 84

Popliteal   129f
Portal   77f, 78f, 83f, 90
Pulmonary   66, 67
Renal   70f, 74, 75, 81, 86
Retromandibular   22, 25, 26
Right brachiocephalic   46, 47, 59, 65
Right hepatic   63, 72, 73, 79, 84
Right portal   73, 81
Right pulmonary   67
Right renal   75

Small saphenous   129f
Splenic   70f, 73-75, 77f, 81, 88f
Subclavian   70f
Superior mesenteric   70f, 75-77f, 82, 87, 88f
Tibial   129f
Vertebral arch   36
Vertebral artery   18-20f, 26, 70f
Vertebral body   35-44
Vocal cord   24, 27

W

Willis 動脈輪   20f, 32f

Y

Yellow ligament   35-37, 39-41

● 編著者プロフィール

似鳥 俊明(にたとり・としあき)
岩手県陸前高田市出身。
岩手医科大学卒業。
杏林大学医学部・放射線科 前教授。

佐々木 康夫(ささき・やすお)
岩手医科大学卒業。
岩手県立中央病院・放射線診断科長。

CT・MRI 解体新書 ─正常解剖─

2012年 1月 1日 第1版
2015年 4月 1日 第1版2刷
2016年10月 1日 第1版3刷
2017年11月 1日 第1版4刷
2020年 4月15日 第1版5刷

編　著	似鳥 俊明、佐々木 康夫
発行者	稲田 誠二
発行所	株式会社 リブロ・サイエンス
	〒163-8510　東京都新宿区西新宿2-3-3
	KDDIビル アネックス2階
	電話 (03) 5326-9788
印　刷	株式会社 ルナテック
表紙デザイン	伊藤 康広(松生庵文庫)

ⒸNITATORI Toshiaki, 2012
ISBN978-4-902496-40-6
Printed in Japan

落丁・乱丁は小社宛にお送り下さい。
送料小社負担にてお取り替えいたします。
定価はカバーに表示してあります。